From O
EXTRAORDINARY

How to Succeed in the Gym by Following
My Four Basic Principals of Fitness

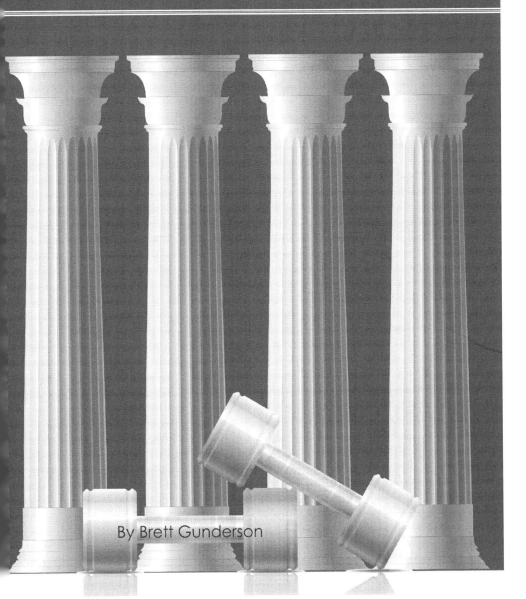

By Brett Gunderson

From Ordinary to Extraordinary: How to Succeed in the Gym by Following
My Four Basic Principals
Copyright © 2015 by Brett Gunderson

For more information, please visit www.elitefitnessoc.com.

Printed in the United States of America
First Edition: (April 2015)

Testimonials

"I first met Gunner about 10 years ago when I moved into the Colony at Fashion Island. I saw him in the gym doing a personal training session with another resident and was impressed with his knowledge as well as his warm personality. His client went on to rave about the great results he was getting with Gunner—and this was after having worked unsuccessfully with numerous trainers before him.

Now, many years later, I have to thank Gunner for the tremendous impact he's had on my life. His expertise is second to none. With his guidance in both exercise and nutrition, I can honestly say I'm in the very best shape of my life at 57 years old! My strength, endurance and energy are up while my body fat is as low as my teenage years. More than that, Gunner's positive energy helps make everyday a better day.

If you're looking to become your very best, and looking for the 'best of the best' in personal training, look no further than Brett Gunderson."

–Dennis Walsh
Resident at The Colony at Fashion Island, Newport Beach, Calif.

*"Training is not an option—it is a **must** for your health, state of mind, bone mass and strength. When facing a health issue, you will get through it twice as fast and heal faster if you have a training program in place. I am 62 years old and will be training for the rest of my life. It has allowed me to have a great quality of life—and that is a value that far surpasses just 'the way you look'…although that is the bonus that comes with it. Elite Fitness is a must for me, and I have tried them all. They are the best in the business and recognize that not everyone and everyday is the same. They work with you, for you and customize each session just for you. I believe every minute I spend with them on my health and overall fitness is what every 'body' needs and deserves to actually live your life in style!"*

–Cynda Lancaster

"I am a single mother of two and have had the pleasure of getting personal training from Elite Fitness. I explained what my goal was and they went above and beyond to help me attain it. With a diet plan and workout program they put together to fit me and my lifestyle, I've hit my goals in under three months. With top-of-the-line equipment and Brett's background, reaching your goals couldn't be easier. This was my first time working out with a personal trainer and I can say it has been a blast. Thanks, Brett, and everyone at Elite Fitness."

–Michelle M.

(continued)

"I would highly recommend Elite Fitness for individuals of all ages who are in need of a personal trainer to provide expert instruction and fitness assistance.

First impressions are important. When first introduced to Elite Fitness, I was immediately impressed with the client-friendly atmosphere provided by owner, Brett Gunderson, and equally impressed with the clean condition of the training facility and excellent, state-of-the-art equipment.

I was instantly put at ease when talking with Brett about a training program that accommodated a 58-years-'young' baby boomer who wanted to tone up, lose weight and lower her blood pressure.

Brett became my personal trainer about 10 weeks ago. I am very happy with the results of my training, as I have lost 15 lbs., lowered my blood pressure and can walk in the hills of Anaheim without gasping for air. I look forward to continuing my training and improving my physical stamina.

Brett is highly skilled, knowledgeable and professional in his interaction with clients. The gym is not crowded and the attentions to detail in the training sessions make an hour fly by quickly.

I generally do not give testimony, but I am so impressed that I want others to enjoy the same quality of personal training I have received. Thank you, Brett, for providing such a valuable service."

–Linda Robinson
Anaheim, Calif.

Acknowledgements

First, to my family: I would like to thank my parents for always being there for me—for supporting me not only through my bodybuilding, but through all of the ups and downs of my life (hopefully, it's a lot more ups now). Words can't describe all you have sacrificed and given to make my life better. To my wife, April, who has always trusted and believed in me. Living with a bodybuilder isn't always the easiest. She was always a big part of helping me to be my best not only on stage but in my business as well. To my son, Cody, for his patience and understanding while I was working and writing this book.

To my gym family: To all of my training partners who helped me perfect my training style and push me to my limits. Special thanks to Keith Lee, who, with your help, we perfected my diet program to get me in the best shape possible. You were always at every show to not only encourage me, but also to make sure I was on-point with every shot. We won together, and I couldn't have done it without you. You'll always be a big part of my life! To Shawn Ray, who took the time to teach me how to pose and be mentally focused and ready for every show. I was so blessed to have so many knowledgeable people help and teach me. Without all of you, I wouldn't have had my foundation to develop my training styles and techniques I use today. To Chris Lund, international photographer and editor of Flex Magazine, for giving me multiple photo shoots and magazine shoots that I'll have forever to remember my journey.

To Dennis Hurley, whose time and guidance helped me turn my passion into a successful business. You've always been there for me to help me with new ideas, and you inspire me to continue to strive to be the best I can be. To Den, Tre, and all the people who encouraged me to write this book: Without your support, this wouldn't have happened. To Susanne Dwyer, who took my words and used her editing skills to make this book a reality.

Thank you to Josh from True Fitness in Fullerton, Calif., for the use of your gym for all of our pictures.

Thank you to everyone in my life—may we continue to make each other better through friendship and love!

Author Bio

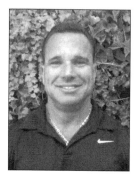

Brett Gunderson grew up in Orange County Calif. He has now lived in Placentia for the past 17 years. He is married to his wife, April, of 15 years. They have one son, Cody, age 9.

He earned his B.S. in kinesiology at CSUF. He returned to CSUF to complete his masters in exercise physiology. His thesis work was done in the gerontology department, studying the benefits and efficiency of strength training with people over the age of 65. It was during this time that Brett perfected his unique style of training. Although Brett has trained professional athletes from three different sports and an Olympic gold medalist, it was his time in the gerontology center that his passion grew to help people rehabilitate from injuries, get their strength and independence back, and improve their quality of life. These were the areas that interested him the most.

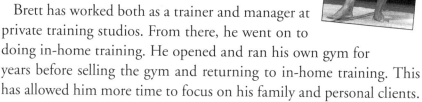

Brett has worked both as a trainer and manager at private training studios. From there, he went on to doing in-home training. He opened and ran his own gym for years before selling the gym and returning to in-home training. This has allowed him more time to focus on his family and personal clients.

Brett developed the "Stay Strong, Live Long" curriculum for the Cordelia Knott Center for Wellness. This strength program focused on muscle recovery, stamina and flexibility for post-cancer and rehab clients. Brett continues to work as a consultant for apartment communities and homeowner associations on equipment purchases and gym layouts. He also provides fitness and nutrition seminars for them.

Brett competed in power lifting and then bodybuilding, winning county and state titles, and competed nationally before retiring from the sport. He still works with competitors on their nutrition and posing routines. He has been featured in a number of fitness magazines.

Foreword

We now look forward to our annual "Fitness Competition," during which we all see great changes in only eight short weeks. Follow the plans set out in this book. You won't regret it.

Once there was a man who found himself in a dark forest surrounded by thick trees and strange sounds. He felt his way forward with his arms outstretched. Often he would trip over a log or step into a hole. After a time, he was scratched and bruised and still saw no end to his dilemma.

Have you ever felt like this when you entered a gym to begin a new workout program? Strange, complicated equipment is everywhere. There are strange sights and sounds. To many, this is a daunting experience. This was my experience seven years ago when I embarked upon my first weight-loss and fitness program. Since then, it has grown into a program for my entire law office. Everyone wanted to get involved. Everyone saw fantastic results. What made the difference? Knowledge. This came from a reliable and motivating source in the person of Brett Gunderson. Brett taught us why we were doing what we did. He taught us the science.

–West Seegmiller
Founder, The Seegmiller Law Firm
Newport Beach, Calif.

From Ordinary to
EXTRAORDINARY
How to Succeed in the Gym by Following
My Four Basic Principals of Fitness

Introduction

For years, I've been asked when was I going to write a book or produce a video on training. My first response was, "Really? Another book on training among the thousands already out there?" Most of these books and videos give you magic promises based on gimmicks or fads meant to make money—and they rarely really help the average individual. That's just not what I do, nor who I am.

For over 25 years, it has been my life's work to make a difference in people's lives by helping them live healthy, active and happy lifestyles. So what changed my mind to the point that I felt compelled to write this book? Since I sold my personal training gym and went back to doing in-home training, I've also gone back into the big-box gyms to train myself. In doing this, I noticed three huge problems that stand out almost every time. The biggest is watching other people train who are either doing the exercise completely wrong or they're doing them almost correctly, but with a little correction on their form, they would achieve far greater results.

The second thing that stands out is how many people come up to me wanting me to help them with their training. Now, if these were your average people, that would be fine, but these are people who have been training for years. Most people would think they really understood training. Most people who are training haven't had the education and experiences I've been privileged to have. How could they understand the "what" and "why" of how to train properly?

How did they learn what they know, and how can they know if they've never been exposed to the types of training I've had?

Of course they're not sure, as they've never been taught what I was taught. Even though I went through a B.S. and a M.S. in exercise physiology that gave me the understanding of how and why the body and muscles work, the answers really lead back to the days when I first started training. Wow, the gyms I went to definitely were not your average gyms. They were hard-core, bodybuilding and power-lifting gyms. Gyms like that just aren't around anymore.

The first gym I went to at the age of 16 was Needham's Gym. It was an old warehouse building with no air-conditioning, no pool, no basketball court and definitely no cardio room or classes. What it did have was lifting chalk flying around and loud voices piercing through the air—an air that was electrifying with an atmosphere I'd never experienced before. Inside, the gym was full of giant men out of a Conan adventure film. They happened to be some of the best bodybuilders and power lifters in the world. Right away, I knew this was the place to be.

Being only 16 years old, I kept my head down and just trained as hard as I could while watching the professionals train. Once they saw that I was coming every day and pushing myself as hard as I could, they began to open up to me. They would ask me to train with them or they would help me out with my training routine. It would be like going to a pro-football game and having the players ask you to come practice with them. I was let in to their inner circle—to be a part of the whole experience. What a time! I soaked up everything I could possibly learn from them. As I look back now, I realize how blessed I was to have grown up in an environment like that.

From that gym, I went on to another gym that had the same atmosphere, but mostly with top bodybuilders and not the power lifters. (By this time, I had realized the problems and injuries that are common with power lifting). I was able to train with many top pro and amateur bodybuilders, always learning more and combining what I'd learned from all of them, eventually developing my own methods and techniques of training based on their fundamentals and what I was learning from my college courses in exercise physiology.

So, back to the second question, of course they don't know all the ins and outs of training. How could they? They have never been around it, let alone grown up and lived it every day. Now, we seem to live in an era of misinformation and intentional misguidance by the fitness industry in order to sell more products, supplements, fad diets and workouts to make more money rather than trying to help people get into better shape and live better lives.

The third problem I noticed was during the time I owned my training studio. About half of the people who were beginners and coming into my training facility were overwhelmed with the equipment and unsure if they were able to do a training program to help them reach their goals. I quickly reassured them that a qualified trainer would be with them at all times and I'd simply explain what they would be required to do and the methods and reasons as to why we train like we do. This would help put them at ease and reassure them that they would succeed in achieving their goals.

Again, I thought, "This is a small studio. How must most beginners, or anyone, feel when they're walking into a huge gym with all that equipment and machines everywhere?" Reflecting on those questions and realizing that I've been extremely blessed with all this knowledge about fitness training and being able to put together training programs—plus having had so many experienced people along the way who helped me reach all my goals—I felt compelled to do the following:

▸ Share what I have learned with others
▸ Help the average person learn how to put together his/her own training program
▸ Teach people the basics of training on every level to be successful in reaching their fitness goals
▸ Help people reach and experience the life they want to live: a life of heath and quality to be able to do all the things they want to enjoy.

How to Go from **Ordinary** *to* **EXTRAORDINARY...**

It's as simple as putting the right rules together and understanding your personal fitness program.

The Four Rules to reaching your fitness goals are:
- No. 1: Consistency
- No. 2: Mentally focusing on the muscle—not on the weight
- No. 3: Proper Form
- No. 4: Muscle Fatigue

By understanding these four concepts, there are no limits and no goals you can't reach. We will go over them in detail and **put you on your way to creating a successful fitness program custom-tailored around you!**

We will also cover all the basics of putting together a fitness program, starting with the basics and breaking down every part so you will understand exactly *how* to do everything and also *why* you are doing it. It's my personal opinion that the more you understand why you're doing what you're doing, the more likely you are to keep doing it and being successful.

These are some of the topics that will be covered:
- How many days to train, both with weights and cardio
- How to properly prepare each daily workout
- What are the best exercises to do, and how to properly do them
- How many exercises to do for each muscle
- How many sets to do for each exercise
- How many reps to do for each set
- How much rest between sets, exercises, muscles and days is best
- What's the best way to put a cardio plan together and what to use to do it
- How to eat for a healthy lifestyle
- Factors to put in place to be successful

My main goal of writing this book is to help anyone walk into a gym feeling confident that they know what to do and how to do it—to give them the confidence to succeed and take out the fear and intimidation of going into a big gym. I also want people to understand the "what" and "why" of their training program—to give them the tools they need to create their own training program, and to help them continue to improve on their fitness no matter what their goals are. Anyone can do this if they choose to—it's not that hard. It really breaks down to many common-sense concepts that you will easily understand and a commitment to following them. Remember, it will be easy to learn and understand all of my methods and techniques, but it's not always as easy to follow them, as there are hidden traps that are easy to fall into. I will teach you how to avoid these traps.

Chapter 1

The Problem

I think we can agree that almost everyone wants to look and feel better. You can't watch television or be on the internet without continuously seeing ads for weight loss, muscle gain, and special foods or supplements you need to take in order to look and feel better. We're constantly seeing what workouts celebrities are doing or the newest diet and/or workout fad of the moment. If any one of these really worked, everyone would be doing it and no more new products would be needed.

It is estimated by the U.S. Weight Loss and Diet Control Market that consumers will spend over $60 billion this year on related nutritional and fitness products. These companies are making more money than ever, yet our nation has become more obese and more confused than ever before.

Research tells us that 75 million Americans will start and fail a new diet four separate times this year. According to the Fitness Industry Association, 45 million Americans have a gym membership, but within 24 weeks of starting, most have already stopped going. There is an obvious problem with these numbers. It's easy to see why people are so confused about eating and training because there is so much misinformation out there. The big companies love that because they know you'll try the latest and greatest new product and they'll gladly take your money. The bad news is there's no magic pill or diet that's going to solve your fitness or weight problems. The good news is **I will give you the knowledge to build and design your workout program and the ability to go into any gym with confidence to perform the exercises with proper form and technique for you to reach your fitness goals**. Once you've learned my basic, standard approach, it's up to you to hit the gym and get in shape. It will take some time and effort, but it will be well worth it. It may be the single greatest investment you make in yourself. It can give you the confidence to do all the things in life you enjoy doing and want to continue doing throughout your lifetime.

Another reason why I wanted to write this book was to answer all of the fitness and nutrition questions that I was continuously asked. Several times each week, people would ask me how to train or eat properly. Now, if these were people who didn't train, I would understand, because the information that's out there is not only confusing but also contradictory. But most of the questions were from people who had been training for years—those whom the average person would think had all the knowledge!

I would start by asking them to tell me about their training program. After hearing their answers, I would ask them, "Why are you training like that?" These are the responses I would get: "That's what someone told me to do;" "That's what I saw someone else do;" "I read it in a magazine or saw it online;" and "That's what I've always done." They had no idea of the what, or why, of their training program. If I had a health problem, I wouldn't ask someone who's healthy about it; I'm going to a doctor to get a professional opinion.

As far as the magazine articles go, I've done a number of magazine photo shoots and have been a part of many more—and they're not telling the truth of what that person is really doing. The photographer takes the pictures of the exercises he's told to take, and a writer somewhere in an office cubicle will put words into workout programs for those pictures. They'll use the same photo shoot for a year's worth of pictures, workout routines and stories. I give them credit for continually coming up with new things to say about the same pictures. So then, what do I tell people that ask for my advice? I tell them the basics that I teach all of my clients from day one: **There are four rules to follow that will build the foundation of your training program and that you will always have in place. These rules will help you reach all your fitness goals. First, however, we need to start from the beginning—and the beginning is getting started or restarted on your fitness program.**

Chapter 2

Getting Started

Sometimes the toughest part of a fitness program is getting started or restarted. You need to have a program to follow and the desire to understand your program. Your program is like a road map: You wouldn't just jump in a car and drive to a place you've never been without looking up the directions, so why would you do that with a fitness program? I will help you lay out your road map to get from point A to point B the fastest and safest way possible. We'll set road markers (goals) to keep you motivated and moving in the right direction.

The first two questions you need to ask yourself are:
1. **What's my motivation?**
2. **What's my final outcome from my fitness program?**

It will be best if you write these down so you have a constant reminder of the reasons you're doing this. There are many different reasons for beginning a fitness program, but they all will follow the same methods and techniques that I will lay out for you.

I got started in an odd way. Although I was an only child, I had a "big brother," Greg Petersen, who lived next door to me. He was five years older than me and did everything a big brother does. He would beat me up constantly, but also protect me from anyone and everyone. He taught me how to play every sport I know, and then showed me he could dominate me in every one as well. Even though I would lose every game, I loved it. It taught me to never give up and to keep trying harder. It made me better in sports and in life.

One day, when he was done with football practice, he decided he would force me to lift weights in his backyard. It seemed odd to me; I wanted to play football or basketball. He said, "You've got to be stronger if you're going to try to beat me." Little did I know that that day would be a day that would forever change the course of my life.

A few weeks later, he sold me his bench press and weight set for

$5.00. I was in sixth grade at the time. Not really knowing what I was doing, I'd do three sets of bench presses every day before school. It did not take long for me to get a little stronger as every week went by. Then came the day that I had my first life-changing moment. We would play baseball every day in school and only one person had ever hit the ball over the wall for a home run. He was the biggest kid in class. I was one of the shortest kids in my class. Then, on that fateful day we were playing, I was up at bat and, feeling stronger, I took a big swing at the ball. I can still remember it flying off the bat and sailing through the air and over the wall into the houses. Everyone was shocked that it was me who had smashed that home run, and I was hooked! Being a smaller kid, this was my way to not only compete with the bigger kids, but to win! From that day on, I rarely missed a day of training. I had all the motivation I needed from that experience.

Looking and feeling better are good motivators, but finding more specific ones, such as fitting into an old dress or being able to do a certain activity, are just as important. Common motivators I hear from my clients are wanting to live active lifestyles throughout their entire lives, being able to travel, playing with grandkids, and staying independent. Unfortunately, I've heard too many stories of people who have been very successful in their business, but neglected their health and fitness to a point whereby they struggle to get through the day-to-day tasks of living. Most of these situations could have been completely avoided with proper exercise and nutrition.

I work with a client who does wealth management, and we talk to his clients about the importance of staying healthy—and not only the physical ramifications of declining strength and mobility, but also the rising costs of health care or in-home care they could need if their problems weren't resolved.

One great example was a client who gave his older parents three months of training to help them get in better physical shape. They were somewhat apprehensive about the training, but decided to take the free sessions. They weren't sure if they could do it or if the sessions would really help them at their age (70+). After about six weeks, they noticed improvements not only in strength and mobility, but also in energy and just plain feeling better.

After the three months were up, they somewhat reluctantly agreed to continue because they thought the price was high. Then came that breakthrough moment for them. In addition to being proud of his new biceps that he would gladly show off to anyone who would listen about his training, he and his wife had to get a physical to renew their life insurance policy. With their new and improved physical bodies, their monthly premiums dropped. In fact, they dropped enough that it more than covered my training expense. His only complaint was that he didn't start training earlier—and now, he was the only one of his friends who could walk the golf course!

You would think all of his golfing friends would be knocking down my door to get in the same shape as he was in, but their reasons were that it would be too much work or take too much time, or they feared they might get hurt or just not be able to do it. All of these excuses are easily shot down when I explain how my clients train two to three days a week. We start at their current ability level, and I never have them do anything I know they can't. We start slowly and consistently push forward, and I explain that it's worth it to at least try for a month. If it's not working, they can stop, but I have never had it not work.

When it comes to getting started, one analogy I love to give people on both training and eating is that it's like running a marathon. Many people who have never run a marathon take up that goal. If you're new to a running program, you don't start out by running 26 miles the first day. That would be insane. Everyone would agree that's ridiculous, yet that's exactly what most people do when they start a diet and exercise program. They're at zero and start at 60 miles an hour. It's easy to see why most people give up so easily with that approach. I tell them that just like someone running a marathon for the first time, run to your ability that first day. It may only be a half–mile, or maybe three miles, but that's your starting point and you keep increasing your distance and speed as you go. It's the same theory with eating and training. Again, that's a pretty easy concept to understand, but most people choose not to follow it.

Start with where you're at and slowly, but continually, keep progressing forward, eating better every week and training a little harder every week. It's not how much body fat you lose in the first week or how strong you are; it's how safely and efficiently you're improving from month to month. With this approach, you'll have a completely changed body and lifestyle that will become easy to maintain. Do set goals, but don't set dates by which to hit your goals. Everyone's body is different and will react differently. Don't compare yourself to anyone but yourself. Stay on track and you'll keep hitting your goals.

Another important lesson I learned came before I was even competing. Most people did 10- to 14-week diets, and I'd see them struggling with almost every aspect of their program. I could see they were trying to do too much, too fast, and they really struggled. When I started getting ready for my first show, I was determined to not let that happen to me. I began my program 24 weeks out from my show and started off by actually increasing my food intake, but only eating "clean" food—no junk. I slowly began to lose weight even though I was eating more food. As each week went by, I would make a little change to my food and cardio plan, but rarely ever noticed much of a difference. By the time I was 12 weeks out (when most people were just getting started), I was ahead of where I needed to be and I really didn't even feel like I was dieting. Although that would change as I got closer to my show—and the changes became more extreme—my body and mind were able to handle it much easier because I was already adjusted to what I was doing and none of the changes were very dramatic. I was making little changes over a long time rather than big changes over a short time.

Now that you know why you're starting a fitness program, write down your final goal and then think about where you're at right now and set some easy goals to accomplish over the first few weeks and months. Having small successes will keep you motivated and on track for your long-term goals. If things get hard, look back at the goals you've accomplished and see how far you've come—and let those successes motivate you.

Chapter 3

Setting Your Goals and Expectations

First, set your long-term goal, which will be your final outcome goal. I don't put time limits on your goals because everybody is different. We all have different genetics and body types, so you have to make realistic goals for yourself. For some people, results come a little faster, and for some, a little slower. What matters are your results—and that your results keep coming!

Remember that it's not just hard work, but hard work that's done efficiently and effectively, that counts. Training hard without proper form and technique will only get you so far. That's one big pitfall I see all the time, everywhere I go.

Fitness is one arena that's different from many others. That's why we have so many different products and diet fads out there. They make wild claims, knowing that if you just start an eating or training program and train hard—but do everything incorrectly—you will still see some benefits from it just because you're doing more than you had been do-ing. The problem is that after about three months, your results will stop, your joints and tendons will become sore, and you will have developed bad habits that will be tough to break. Or if you're following some crazy diet fad, again, you're taking in less calories than you were before, therefore, you will see some quick results, but they don't last, and what they don't tell you is that 50 percent of the initial weight loss is water weight, not fat weight. Once you go back to eating as you normally had, the weight comes right back on, so you become frustrated and look for the next new thing. That's what all the companies are planning on because they already have the next "latest and greatest" product to sell you. Think about it: If there were a perfect product or diet fad, everyone would be in shape and there would be no need for any more products. Looking back over the last 60 years, who has always been able to get into shape? Answer: bodybuilders! Do they have the secret? Yes, but it's not really a secret; it's training and eating properly, while being consistent at doing both.

You need to have an open mind to change and you need to reestablish a "new normal" that will change your body and your lifestyle.

One of the best pieces of advice I got when I was bodybuilding was to not think about or compare myself to anyone else. It doesn't matter how someone else looks; that would only be a negative mindset. Instead, I focus only on myself and my body and make it the best I possibly can. This actually took a lot of pressure off me, and **my goal was to be the best me I could be.** The only comparisons I made were: Did I look the best I could for this year, and second, is that better than last year? If I could answer "yes" to both of those questions, I felt that I had won, regardless of where the judges might have placed me.

With your long-term goal in place, go back to the beginning and start with some short-term goals. These may be as simple as, "I'm going to train three times this week." Plan out the time for each day you're going to train, and make it an appointment. This will make it more likely for you to follow though with each session.

Next, set some goals for the month, such as, "I'm not going to miss any training days," or "I'm going to do five more minutes of cardio each session," or "I'm going to increase the intensity of my training a little more." All of these shorter-term goals will help you stay focused to reach your end goal. Have a couple of midway goals, as well, such as dropping a dress size or belt loop, seeing more definition in your muscles, or noticing that you feel better and have more energy than before. Remember how you felt when you started so you can compare that to how you feel at different points in your program.

I don't like to use weight loss as a goal for the following reason: I've seen many clients lose 20 pounds of fat and put on 12 pounds of muscle over three to four months. They've completely changed how their bodies look and have hit their goals, but on the scale, it's only an eight-pound difference, when, in actuality, it's a 32-pound difference. **Remember, clothes and mirrors don't lie; they give you better feedback than a scale.**

I had one client who wanted to lose over 100 pounds. We set his short-, medium- and long-term goals and began knocking off one goal at a time. He started losing inches and dropping belt loops. He used his belt to remind him of where he had started and where he was now. Before long, he was at the smallest belt hole—and even that was getting too big. Rather than get a smaller belt, he took a leather punch and put in a new hole. Then it was another hole and then another. It was his constant reminder of where he used to be and where he was going. After a while—and after about six newly made leather punches—he had to tuck the belt into his pants. Before the year was over, he had lost 120 pounds and had hit his goals along with becoming stronger and having more muscle and energy than ever before. Now, that belt hangs on his wall as a constant reminder of what he accomplished.

When you hit a few small goals or a medium goal, give yourself a reward—but not a cheat meal! Today, we seem to always reward ourselves with bad food or alcohol. You need to have a different mindset. Think of things you like to do and make it fun. It doesn't have to be food! Make it something fun and enjoy your success!

That brings us to another topic: What do you do once you've hit your end goal? How many times have we seen someone work so hard for so long and hit his/her end goal only to free fall backward? How does this happen? Unfortunately, it can happen very easily. The good news is that it can also be prevented fairly easily. Once you hit your final goal, there was all the blood, sweat and tears that went into chasing that goal. Wow! You've done it! You're there! This actually can be a dangerous place to be in if you don't have a maintenance or lifestyle goal in place. The reason is you feel like you're done. You're going to be excited and have a great sense of accomplishment—and you should. You've worked very hard to get where you are. One problem is that at this point, most people become complacent because they've done it; it's over. The big mistake they make is they don't have a lifestyle goal in place. You need to reset your goals, refocus and stay motivated.

Your goal after your end goal is to stay in the shape you're in. This goal will be much easier to maintain with the right strategies in place. You're already there physically, but you need to continue to stay there mentally. It's easy to have a bit of a let down.

I personally experienced this, and truthfully, it was harder than I ever could have imagined. I was 37 years old and at the top of my game in bodybuilding. I was stronger and bigger than ever before and set to place in the top five at the Mr. USA the following year. I had already passed my end goal of winning the super heavyweight class at the Mr. California and had done multiple magazine photo shoots. I'd gone farther in bodybuilding than I or anyone else could have imagined. But in order to focus more on my family and business, I decided to retire from competitive bodybuilding.

All my life, I couldn't wait to get to the gym to try to out-train anyone and everyone. Even after a show, I was already excited to get back in the gym, train and prepare to be even better for next year. When it was over, I made the mistake of not having a lifestyle goal set for myself. Honestly, I had never even thought about it. That's the mistake that created the problem for me. All at once, there were no more goals to chase. I realized there would be no more magazine photo shoots to prepare for, no more trophies to get or hand out at other shows. I wouldn't be asked to attend grand openings of nutrition stores; there wouldn't be any more sponsors or buzz about my next show. That part of my life was over. All of these goals and dreams I'd chased all my life and had accomplished were gone with that one decision. I thought to myself, "How do I get motivated to work hard at the gym now that all the goals I've been chasing all my life are done, and I'm not going to be training at that extreme level anymore?" I thought to myself, "How do I get motivated to train when I'm not going to be trying to train at that level and with no goal in front of me?" Honestly, I had days of doubt, wondering if it was worth it to even keep training. I knew the importance of fitness training and staying healthy, so quitting was never really an option for me. I needed an answer to the new question of what was my new lifestyle goal. I needed to redefine my goals for myself and for my new lifestyle. Using my own techniques and philosophy of training, I designed my workouts to challenge myself in a different way. My philosophy would stay the same, but the style of training would change to not only fit my new lifestyle, but also to keep me mentally focused.

Once you've hit your end goal, it's extremely important—especially if it's weight that you've lost—to maintain that weight for six months.

This will help your body reestablish its new set point. Once you've done this, you're likely to not only keep the body you have now, but constantly keep making minor improvements along the way. Maintaining this new fitness level will be easier, as you've already done all the hard work. All that work and dedication has made your body more efficient, and it will now want to stay that way.

Back to the marathon runner: Once he/she can run 26 miles regularly, then how easy will it be to run 10-15 miles and have fun mixing up the intensity or style to keep his/her body guessing what they're doing while still improving at the same time—but not killing themselves with 26-mile runs all the time?

Chapter 4

The Rules of Strength Training
Rule No. 1: Consistency

I f you want success, you have to be consistent! A good friend told me one time that if you just show up on time and work hard, you'll already be ahead of 90 percent of the other people out there. If time is a factor or you're tired, modify your workout to make it easier. Just get it in and don't skip a training session. Chances are, you'll end up having a better session than you thought and it will put you in a better position for your next workout. The same thing goes with eating. Try to stick to your meal plan the best you can, but if you completely blow it, don't beat yourself up over it. Let it go and make sure for your next meal, you're back on track. As you become more consistent, it will be easier for you to stay consistent. As you reach each goal, this will help motivate you to become more consistent. This is an area in which everyone could use some help. Plan your training times; if possible, have a workout partner. Tell people what you're trying to do. These things will help you to be held more accountable to yourself and to others. Stay focused on your goal(s). If you get support from family and friends, they will help you get through the tough times— and hitting your goals is always more fun to celebrate with the people who have stood behind you and supported you along the way. After you've been going to the same gym at the same time for a while, you'll make new friends. They will also help motivate you on your journey to reaching your goals.

Along my journey, I had great training partners who would always push me to bring out my best. I had a great friend who would help me get ready for my competitions. I had a tendency to not see myself as I really looked. I would think others looked better than I did on stage, and one time, my friend grabbed me as soon as I got off stage. It was my second year competing. He took me backstage, where there was a tape playing of the show. I can still remember him saying, "Look at that! Do you see that? That's *you* up there and that's how you really look!" Now, when you go back out there, act like the winner you are! I saw everything in a brand-new light. Wow, did that motivate me! I still remember looking at the TV monitor and thinking, "Is that really me up there?" That's why I encourage people to take pictures throughout their fitness journey. It's hard to see the constant results because they are happening slowly. And you see yourself everyday, so it's hard to see the little changes that are happening all the time.

Chapter 5

The Rules of Strength Training
Rule No. 2: It's All in the Mind!

I can't emphasize the following enough, as every rep, set and exercise will depend on your getting this concept down: **You will need to use your brain as much as your muscles when training!**
This is the biggest rule to follow—and the rule that's broken most of the time by everyone.

YOUR FOCUS IS ON THE MUSCLE YOU'RE TRAINING— NOT ON THE WEIGHT YOU'RE LIFTING!

Again, I can't emphasize this enough! We've all done it. How much can we lift? And all your focus is on the weight, but you're not focused on the muscle you're training. What happens then is the muscle isn't being used to its fullest capacity. It's easy to lose form, and the efficacy of the exercise just drops way down and the risk of other muscles taking over goes up. Also, your risk of injury will be much higher. This is easy to understand, but hard to put into practice. It will take a lot of patience and practice to perfect this. Once you do, however, the results will be incredible.

When I work with people who have been training for a long time and get them to switch over to my methods of focusing on the muscle, I usually get the same two responses every time: "Wow, I've never felt my muscles like that before" and "I could feel it all the way to the bone." The reason is they are able to isolate each muscle and completely fatigue it, making it the most efficient and productive way to train. This will help you get fast and safe results.

The easiest example to show this is using an arm curl. Take a medium amount of weight and lift it 10 times. Now, take the same weight and lift it slowly on the way up, feeling and focusing on your bicep contracting—no swinging or moving any other body parts, just the arms. As you slowly get to the top of the exercise, flex and contract your bicep as hard as you can. (This recruits even more muscle fibers to more completely work the muscle). Now, slowly lower the weight through the same plane of motion, feeling your bicep stretching down to the beginning point of the exercise. Then, with no momentum or swing, slowly repeat the same rep with your mind completely focused on your bicep. I guarantee you will not only feel the difference, but you will understand the reasoning behind this method. The muscle doesn't know how much weight you're lifting—your brain does. You can take that 40-pound barbell curl and, when done properly, it will feel heavier to the muscle than a 70-pound barbell curl done the regular way. This concept is tougher for men to follow because we always want to judge our workout on if we were stronger or lifted more weight, when it should be judged on whether the muscle is as fatigued and pumped as possible. When I switched to this method of training, my strength didn't drop, but the amount of weight I was lifting dropped by about 30 percent because I was now training properly with my focus on my muscle.

Mentally, it was difficult for me to decrease the amount of weight I had been lifting. It was frustrating and humbling to be lifting weight 30 percent lighter and having it feel heavier than ever. But what I was doing wasn't getting me any more results. In fact, it was only making my joints and tendons sore. I was accruing small muscle injuries along the way, and my strength gains had completely stopped. Something had to change. Once I checked my ego at the door and completely bought into this new way of training, my mind and body were changed forever. I used what I was learning at the gym, along with what I was learning in kinesiology at school, and developed what became my basic foundational rules and principles of training. The new workouts, the way my muscles were feeling, and the results were amazing. I was getting the best workouts and results of my life. And by the way, it actually made me stronger. It wasn't too long before I was back lifting the same amount of weight, but now doing it properly—and the results just kept coming. The other thing I noticed was the relief I had in my joints and tendons. When you're focusing on the weight and not on the muscle, it's easy to lose focus and use other muscles and put your joints and tendons under a higher amount of pressure.

Back when I was competing nearly every day, someone would ask me how much I could lift or bench press. Rarely did anyone ever ask *how* I trained to look like that. I would give them my standard answer: "I don't know. I haven't done a flat bench press in over 15 years." They would seem puzzled that I didn't bench press and would walk away most of the time. Somehow, somewhere, the flat bench press became the standard to measure strength. Personally, the reason I don't do a flat bench press is the fact that it puts too much pressure on my shoulders, elbows and bicep tendons. I feel like my chest gets a better workout by using a slight incline for both bar and dumbbell presses. Once you've mastered this rule, you are well on your way to achieving great gains in your fitness program.

Chapter 6

The Rules of Strength Training
Rule No. 3: Proper Form

Proper form goes hand-in-hand with Rule No. 2: focusing on the muscle. Proper form means going though the right plane of movement at the predetermined pace that is set for each rep of each set. It also means having your body in the right position at all times throughout the entire movement. Proper form includes everything from the placement of your feet and hands to the curve of your back and the proper angles of the joints. In chapter 14, I give you both visual and written examples of proper form for the basic exercises for each muscle. This will help you to better understand how to use proper form with each exercise.

When I go into a gym and look around, I'd estimate that more than 80 percent of the people I see training have very poor form. With poor form come all the same problems associated with not having your focus on the muscle. If you're doing an exercise and you can't pinpoint exactly where and how it's working, you're probably doing it wrong. Each exercise should be performed with detailed attention to not only the muscle you're training but to the stretch of the muscle and the contraction of the muscle. This will help you achieve greater gains and also limit the chance of injury because, at all times, you're fully aware of your movement and your strength limitations. Too often, I see people training and I have no idea what muscle they're trying to train.

Through these methods and examples, I will prepare you to go into any gym, feeling confident that you can properly do every exercise and have a better understanding of what you're doing than most every other person in the gym. I don't mean to be hard on people who aren't training properly; actually, I want to help them. It's not their fault they don't understand proper form—no one has ever taught them. I learned from the experts I was able to train with every day of my life while I was growing up and while I was competing. I have this lifetime knowledge base and my main goal is to help pass this knowledge on to as many people as possible to help them reach their fitness goals.

Chapter 7

The Rules of Strength Training
Rule No. 4: Muscle Fatigue

This is the last and final rule, but there isn't an exact level of muscle fatigue I can give you.

The basic rule of muscle fatigue is that once you are no longer able to do another rep with proper form and focus, the set is over. There are different levels of muscle fatigue, and that is what you will have to adjust to reach your personal fitness goals. Now that I'm not competing anymore, I have adjusted my level of predetermined muscle fatigue for myself. For example, when I was competing, I would do an incline bench press with a weight I could successfully perform at least eight times on my own, but then have my spotter help me perform another eight reps. Since I was training for size and had a spotter, I would do as many reps as I could until I could no longer completely control the weight coming down. My spotter would help ease the weight at the bottom of the exercise and assist me in pushing it up while I maintained proper form all the time. If I ever felt that I couldn't completely control the weight on the way down, I wouldn't do another rep. Now that I'm training to stay in shape, I pick a weight I can do 12-20 times, depending on the style I'm using that day, and perform it until I'm not going to be able to lift it again with proper form and control through both planes of motion. Since it's dangerous to do a bar press without a good spotter, I stick to doing dumbbells or a Smith machine so I can go to failure and even get some half reps in the bottom without getting stuck under a bar. Since I'm not getting assisted reps from a spotter, my reps will be higher, and the rest in between sets will be less to help increase intensity and fatigue. Along with less rest, to increase the fatigue factor, I will also drop the amount of weight to help keep my reps high (12-20 range). If you are training to gain size, you will want to find a good training partner to help spot you and get those extra forced reps in. If you're training to improve your muscle structure and get in good shape, you'll train using the example that I'm using now. It would still be a great idea to have a good training partner, as they can assist you with the sets and make sure you're using proper form all the time. A good partner will help motivate you and push you to do your best. They also help with rule No. 1, consistency, because you both will be accountable to each other. It also makes going to the gym more fun when you're doing it together.

These are the four basic rules that make up the foundation of your training program. With this foundation as your base, there are no goals you can't accomplish. These rules will apply to all your weight-training programs regardless of the results you want. There are endless variations of what you can do, but these rules will always be the core of your training program.

Chapter 8

Basic Terminology

1. **Your Training Day:** This is everything you will do on the day you go to the gym.

2. **Strength-Training Exercise:** This is one of the machine, dumbbell(s), bar and/or body movements you will perform.

3. **Sets:** Each exercise will consist of a number of sets, usually 2-4. This is the number of times you perform each exercise.

4. **Repetitions or Reps:** This is the number of times you perform the movement until failure in one set, usually between 12-20 reps for each set.

5. **Rest:** This refers to the time in between training days, muscles trained, exercise and sets performed.

6. **Concentric Movement:** This is the part of the muscle that's being shortened and brought into a flexed position.

7. **Eccentric Movement:** This is when the muscle is stretching or lengthening.

8. **The Transition:** This is the critical part of each rep between moving from the concentric movement to the eccentric movement or vise versa.

9. **Pause Rep:** This is where you would pause (stop) the movement of the rep between the transitional point of the rep without relaxing the muscle.

10. **Half Rep:** This is when you would only go halfway through a rep and pause at the halfway point and hold for 1-5 seconds. Half Reps can be done on either part of the concentric or eccentric movement, dependent on the exercise.

11. **Speed Count:** This is the length of time during a rep, half rep or set.

12. **Drop Set:** This is when the first working set is completed, you immediately lower the amount of weight and begin another set. When that set is done, you will repeat the same process. Drop sets usually contain 2-4 sets.

13. **Superset:** This is when you perform one exercise and immediately go to another exercise and perform that one. That is one superset. Then the same sequence will be performed again. Supersets can be done working the same muscle or two different muscles at once.

14. **Giant Set:** This is the same as a superset, only adding one or two more exercises to it.

15. **Circuit Set:** This is performed with light weight and done by combining multiple exercises (8-15), moving from one exercise to another with very little rest, usually working multiple body parts, if not the entire body.

Chapter 9

Reps Defined and Explained

The most frequently asked question I get from people is, "How many reps should I do?" **The number of reps will depend on your intended outcome of training.**

Let's take some time to clear up a few things right now. I know most of you have heard—and it does sound good—that the heavier you lift, the more your size will increase. The other misconception is that if you want to lean out, you need to do a higher number of reps. If you only want to be stronger, and strength is your main goal, then, yes, you lift heavy. This is why many athletes lift heavy because they don't want to get much bigger and lose flexibility and speed. They're training for strength and speed. Lifting with low reps (3-8) is great for strength gains, but not conducive to improving muscle quality and the overall physique most people are looking for.

It's extremely rare to see a power lifter that's in great shape. There is no way you can fatigue a muscle with reps that low. You will run out of the energy to produce the force you need to do more reps, but the muscle will barely be fatigued. For example, if I did any exercise for 5 reps, I could immediately drop the weight by 25 percent and still get another 15-20 reps. Fatigue and muscle exhaustion is what is going to give you the fast and lasting results you want. Again, the level of fatigue you choose will depend on the results you want to achieve (more muscle or toned and sculpted). As to the second misconception, high reps will help you lean out. The only contributing factor that might help a little is the fact that you're probably increasing your heart rate during your training session by using higher reps. Let me be perfectly clear, **you lean out by burning more calories than you take in and by making sure the calories you are taking in are good, clean, nutritionally dense calories that will help your body run more efficiently.** How light the weight is or how many reps you do will have little effect on your body fat.

A "rep" is moving the muscle from the starting point through the full range of the eccentric or concentric contraction and then returning back to the starting point.

Things to avoid while performing your reps:
▸ Do not let the weight take you through the movement.

▸ Do not bounce or swing the weight during the transitional point of the movement.

▸ Avoid over-extending the joint or locking it out (this puts un-needed pressure on the joint and tendon and takes the pressure off the muscle).

Remember, the idea is to fatigue the muscle. When it's fatigued, you don't need to pause or rest in order to get more reps. (By this, I mean do not rest in between reps, but rather, keep the motion going and the pressure on the muscle).

Things to focus on while doing your reps:
▸ The most important is to always be focused on the muscle you're training, going through the right plane of movement, controlling the weight on the negative phase to make the muscle work harder.

▸ Do force a hard contraction at the flex point without locking out. (This will also help keep you focused on the muscle and achieve a fuller fatigue while recruiting more muscle cells to fire).

▸ Always be in control of the weight you're lifting.

▸ On working sets, always perform as many reps as possible while following our basic rules.

Half Reps
Half reps are best done on a machine or with dumbbells. This is another technique to help you further fatigue the muscle for greater results. Once you have performed as many reps as you can, you can add in half reps. From the bottom of the movement, come up halfway and pause the weight for 1-5 seconds, then slowly return and repeat until complete failure. Or do the opposite by coming down halfway, paus-

ing for 1-2 seconds and returning, flexing the muscle and then repeating until failure. I generally prefer the first method. By holding in the halfway position, your muscles will be forced to fully contract at a spot they're normally not used to, which will help with fatigue and increase strength in the muscle.

Warm-up Sets

With my first exercise for each muscle, I will do two warm-up sets. These sets are done with lighter weight and performed slowly with a deep stretch to loosen up the muscles and tendons. I only do 8-15 easy reps that are not done to failure. You don't want to pre-exhaust the muscle before your first working set. They are done to get you ready to start the first working set of the first exercise. After the first working set is done, there's no need to do any more warm-up sets, as the muscles are already warmed up and ready to go. Don't waste time and needless effort on extra sets that aren't going to help you. Extra warm-up sets can actually take away from your working sets, making your workout less effective.

Working Sets

I always like to change up the number of reps I do to keep the muscles guessing and to prevent me from getting in a set routine and becoming complacent. That being said, there are rules and guidelines I follow for many exercises and muscle groups.

Starting with upper-body exercises, my rep range is between 12-20 reps per set, all performed to failure, after doing two warm-up sets on the first exercise. I like to start my training session with one or two power exercises. With these exercises, my rep range will be more around 12-15 for the first two sets, then I'll lower the weight and get closer to 20 reps to increase fatigue. From the power exercises, I will move on to the isolation exercises. With these, there's even more focus on the precision of the movement, and I will want to get in the 16-20 rep range while getting a hard squeeze of the muscle on each contraction. I like to end each muscle group with an exercise in which I will do only one set, or a quick two-set drop, and up my reps to the 25-30 range to completely fatigue the muscle. The weight will be light and I'll start with a slow rep time and gradually increase my rep speed as I feel the muscle fatiguing. From this set, your muscles will reach full fatigue and include a great muscle pump.

Lower Body

All the same techniques from upper body apply to lower body with one big exception: the rep range. Legs have much larger muscles and will not fatigue as easily as the smaller, upper-body muscles. To achieve that same type of fatigue, we need to up our rep range. On the power exercises, it will be 15-25 reps per set, and on the isolation exercises, it will be 20-30 reps per set. This will take more mental determination to get through. It will be more exhausting, and the lactic acid will make the muscles burn. But push through that, as the results will be well worth it. As an added bonus, you will burn many more calories from a hard leg day.

Changing Your Reps

You will still follow the previous rules and examples from before, but you can vary it. One variation is to have a heavier day. You may do more sets in the lower-rep ranges to push some heavier sets. When doing this, you still want to throw in a high-rep set with each exercise. I recommend increasing the reps on the lighter set to 25-30 for upper body and 30-50 for lower body. These sets will be killers, but they will definitely push your muscles to complete fatigue. On lighter days, or days you don't feel you have the extra energy, go with higher reps: 20-plus for upper body and 30-plus for lower body. Cut down on the rest between sets and between exercises and you'll get in a great workout with a phenomenal muscle pump in half the time. It's good to mix things up as much as possible. Now that I know my body so well, I usually don't pre-plan my workout style for the day, but rather, go by how I'm feeling that day. In the beginning, I find it's better to plan out your days so you don't fall into the trap of repeating the same style or technique you like best.

Speed of Your Reps

This is something that will change as you improve and increase your intensity level. To start, I have people do a basic, two-second down and a one-second return for each rep. Once you have the basics down, you can begin to play and experiment with varying the speed of your reps. You will need to use lighter weight in order to hit your rep range. Depending on your speed, your rep range may drop to 8-12. For example, I would use a weight about 30 percent lighter than my normal heavy set in which I'd get around 15 reps, and I'd do a 5-1-3. That's five seconds on the way down, with a one-second pause at the bottom and a three-second return. The first few reps will be easy, but keeping the movement this slow, while getting an extra stretch and hard flex at the top, will begin to fatigue you very quickly. That is why the reps will be a little lower, but you will achieve full fatigue.

The first time I have people do this, they think they're having a weak day because the weight they can normally do 20-plus times, now they're struggling hard to get 10 reps. It's all due to changing the speed. That's a hard example; an easier one would be a 3-2 rep. That's lowering the weight down over a three-second count and returning it over a two-second count. There are many variations you can play with. When performing these types of sets, remember to still throw in your one high rep set at the end of each set. You will be shocked how fast you fatigue with the high rep set. Slowing the speed down will dramatically increase your muscle fatigue.

Review of Reps

If you're not hitting your rep range, the weight is too heavy! Lower it and hit your rep range. **If you're able to go past your rep range, increase your weight, as it's too light and you're not going to stress the muscle enough to make it improve.** At the end of your light-fatigue sets, it's okay to go over your rep range. Go to failure, and if you go 10 over, that's okay. You're going for high reps and full fatigue. Don't hold back. If you don't hit your rep range for the final light set, drop the weight and do it again right away and hit your rep range to reach total fatigue.

Chapter 10

Rest Between Sets and Exercises

There is no exact answer for how long to rest between sets and exercises, but there are many good rules to follow to determine how long you should rest between them.

We'll start with **rest between sets.** One rule to keep in mind is that **you never want to start a set when your breath or oxygen will give out before your muscle fatigues.** Another general rule is **the more taxing the exercise, the more rest you will need between sets.** This usually applies to training bigger muscles, or doing power exercises, as you will also need more rest between each set. Example: You are going to be more out of breath after a leg exercise than after a bicep exercise, and you will be more out of breath after a leg press or squat than after a leg extension or leg curl. You want to make sure you get enough rest to perform the next set to muscle failure. After performing a heavy leg press or squat until failure, you may need 1-2 minutes until you're ready to go again. On the other hand, after a bicep curl, you may only need 10-30 seconds of rest. Although you don't have your breath back, your biceps are ready to go and you won't run out of air because the oxygen demand isn't as high for biceps as it is for leg or back exercises. **The better trained and more in shape you are, the less rest you will need between sets.**

When you're lowering the weight you're using for each set, you will also want to cut down on your rest time. Another example would be if you're doing a chest or shoulder press (both power exercises). You may rest for 45-60 seconds between sets, but when doing chest flies or side laterals for shoulders (both isolation exercises), you might only rest for 20-45 seconds. That's the difference between the power exercises and the isolation exercises. When performing your light-fatigue set at the end, I prefer no rest at all to increase complete muscular fatigue. This means you usually have to drop to a very light weight to hit your high-rep range, but trust me, it won't feel light. It may feel and be harder than your first heavy-working set. You'll have to try different variations to see what works best for you. Remember to keep changing it up to not only shock your muscles, but to help you stay focused on the muscles you're training. You don't want to wait until you have 100 percent of your breath back. You're wasting time if you do that and you're delaying the fatiguing process. Too many times, I'll see people talking, sitting, and wasting time until their next set. That will get you nowhere. Have your plan in your mind of what you're doing now and what the next exercise will be. You can talk and hang out all you want after your training is over.

Rest between exercises: Here, you will want to get to your next exercise as quickly as possible. By the time you get to it and get it ready, you're probably going to be ready to start your first set. Before you start your next exercise, you should have about 90 percent of your breath back, and it's time to hit it again following the same set of rest rules. **On power exercises, you will rest longer than you will when performing isolation exercises.**

Time between sets and exercises gives you more variations to change up your intensity. Once you are adjusting to the basic workouts, try varying the time periods. On heavier days, you may rest a little longer, and on lighter days, you may cut your rest time in half. Cutting your rest time will pick up your intensity. You'll have to go lighter in order to hit your rep range, but the muscle pump and fatigue will be huge. **Remember, it's not about how much weight you're lifting! It's about training the muscle to full fatigue and getting the best results out of what you're doing!**

You've achieved the hardest part by just getting to the gym. Don't blow your workout by wandering around, thinking about what to do next, or stopping to talk to everyone. You're there for one reason and one purpose. **Don't let any distractions ruin your results and your workout.**

Also, if the gym is busy, you need to have a backup plan in mind. When you finish your exercise and you're on to your next exercise, if someone else is on that machine, don't sit around and wait for it. Have one or two backup exercises in mind and get to those. You can come back to that exercise or just replace it with your backup. Wasting time in the gym is like putting a small hole in a balloon. Once the air is out, it's out and it's over. Fully fatiguing the muscle requires your getting through the exercises and sets in the right amount of time, or just like that balloon, you will lose that muscle pump, and the fatigue you're shooting for will be off. I see this happen too often: People are at the gym doing everything but what they should be doing—training!

To help avoid this, know your gym; know your backup exercises and where they are in your gym.

Chapter 11

Number of Sets and Exercises

A gain, there is no perfect number of sets I can tell you to do, although, again, there are guidelines to help you determine the right number of sets for you. I'll outline a simple equation. You just need to follow the guidelines and you'll be fine. Most people don't do the right amount of sets—or fail to do the sets properly—for what they are trying to achieve. I made this mistake for years when I first started training. I was doing more than double the amount of sets I needed to do and not doing them to my fullest potential.

If you're a highly motivated person, this is not only an easy mistake to make, but the reasoning behind it will make sense to you. In business and life, we think the harder we work and the more we do, the better results we will get. Right? Not with training! Again, if you start out training this way, you will get results for a good three months, maybe more. Then your program will fall flat. You will stop progressing. Strength gains will slow or stop, and sometimes even decrease. Your motivation will plummet, and you will have a high risk of injury or tendonitis. This is where you want to work smarter, not harder. I know I just finished preaching about doing every set to failure and sometimes pushing beyond that, but for the total number of sets and exercises, it's different. **When you're training each set to failure and you're completely exhausting the muscle, this creates a different situation for the muscle. You don't need to do as many sets or exercises as you think.** Logically thinking, if you've completely exhausted the muscle, is it possible to exhaust it more? The simple answer is "no!" Could you still do more? Yes, but know you're breaking down the muscle tissue beyond the point for it to improve. You begin to damage the muscle tissue and it's going to struggle to repair and improve. Since you're doing less sets and exercises than before, you can see the need to push every set you do to its limits.

Having trained for over 30 years, I've seen countless people come into the gym everyday and train for 1-2 hours, but yet they haven't changed their bodies at all in the last 3-5 years. I think to myself, "That's crazy." If I were putting that much time and effort into something and not getting results, why keep wasting my time? The truth is, most people do too many sets and too many exercises, BUT they never get the full potential out of any of them. **You don't need to do a lot of volume; what you do need to do is make every set count!**

Back to determining the right amount of sets and exercises for your program. First, you need to know how many days you're going to train per week. By knowing how many days per week you're going to train, you will know what muscles to train and the number of sets and exercises to do. It can be anything from 2-6 days per week depending on your time and your goals.

First, a quick look back on my beginning days as a personal trainer. I think this will help encourage many people just getting started. If you had asked me 25 years ago, "Can a person get good, solid results from training 2-3 times per week for less than an hour?," I would have told you "NO!" I may have even said, "Don't waste your time." Wow, was I wrong—dead wrong! If your goal is to be a competitive bodybuilder, then, yes, you need to train six days a week. If you want to get in great shape and improve your all-around fitness, it can easily be done if you follow the principles I've laid out in this book.

So what changed my mind so convincingly? I saw it happen, not a few times, not half the time, but almost every time over my 25 years of training people. I would train most of my clients 2-3 days per week. The key was they had to follow my techniques and methods of training and eating. Since I was personally training them, the training part was a given. It takes a few weeks for your body to adapt to these methods, but once it does, it's on! Even the people who only saw me twice a week, if they were consistent on making their appointments, they saw amazing results after only 8-10 weeks. The great thing is the results didn't stop; they continued to make improvements. I even had clients who wouldn't push themselves very hard. They would train at 60-70 percent of what I knew they were capable of, yet they still achieved great, lasting results! It all goes back to the methods and rules of how to properly train. Their advantage was not needing to know how to put the reps, sets, exercises and routines together because I did that for them. My goal now is to teach everyone how to put the right training program together so they can get the same results my clients have achieved over the past 25 years.

Bear with me as I give one more example that's close to my heart, and I hope it can motivate some older people who have never trained before to start a training program following my methods. When I was in graduate school for exercise physiology, my thesis project was done in the gerontology department at CSUF. I conducted a strength-training program for people 65 and older who had medical clearance from their doctors. Most of the people (I hate to call them "subjects") never had done any type of strength training; and many of them also had a medical condition, which ranged from heart attacks, strokes, diabetes, broken bones, loss of bone density, and others. For my project, they would train for 45 minutes, two times per week for one semester. We had four different groups with 15-20 people per group. For the first two weeks, saying they didn't like me was an understatement. They were experiencing muscle soreness for the first time, and it was more work than many of them had done in decades. They were more than happy to take out their aches and pains on me! Some of the names they called me and things they said to me, you wouldn't expect out of someone who looked like your grandmother, but I understood what they were going though. The muscle soreness and stiffness, as well as the training itself, weren't fun at first, but I continued to encourage them and tell them it would get easier and they'd be glad they did it. I'm not sure if anyone believed me, but I managed to get them through the first few weeks. After about four weeks, everything changed! Not only were they happy to come to class, but they were excited to see me and tell me what they were able to do. They were doing things they hadn't done in years because they were stronger now. They felt better, both physically and mentally, than they had in years. They said the workouts were easier, but I told them we were actually training harder than ever. Their bodies, muscles and minds had adjusted to the way we were training. Now, instead of being the hated one, I was the loved one. They were so overly appreciative of me that I never forgot it. That's why I absolutely love my work. It doesn't get much better than that—to help people live a higher quality of life both mentally and physically. As for the results of the project, almost everyone's strength improved by approximately 300 percent—some more, a few less—but still a significant difference. If they could do it, you don't have any excuse not to do it.

If you're going to train two days per week, you're going to want to train every muscle on both days. Your guidelines will be to do 2-3 exercises per body part, doing two sets for each exercise. If you're going to train three times per week, I'd recommend splitting the workouts, alternating a leg day, then an upper-body day, and repeat. You'll do three sets per exercise and 2-3 sets per body part. For example, one week you would do legs twice, and the next week, upper body twice, and so on, just alternating legs and upper body.

If you're more advanced and want to train harder for better, faster results, your split will look something like this.

Day 1:
Chest and Shoulders: 3 exercises each, 2-3 sets per exercise

Day 2:
Quads, Hamstrings and Calves: 3 exercises each, 2-3 sets per exercise

Day 3:
Back, Triceps and Biceps: 3 exercises each, 2-3 sets per exercise

This is a basic template to start with. You will adjust and mix things up as you improve, but always follow the basic principles and rules we've laid out. Some days you may add in some extra exercises and/or sets, and some days you may lower the numbers of exercises and sets. You will learn how to "feel out" your body and know when to change it up.

The number of sets in these workouts does not include your two warm-up exercises for the beginning of your training session.

If you're a beginner and are going to train four days per week, this is the plan to follow:

Day 1: Legs
A. *Quads:* 3 exercises (2-3 sets)
B. *Hamstrings:* 2 exercises (2-3 sets)
C. *Calves:* 1-2 exercises (2 sets)

Day 2: Upper Body
A. *Back:* 2 row exercises and 1 pull exercise (2-3 sets)
B. *Chest:* 2 press exercises and 1 fly exercise (2-3 sets)
C. *Shoulders:* 1 press exercise, 1 side lateral, 1 rear lateral, 1 shrug (2-3 sets)
D. *Triceps:* 2 exercises (3 sets each) or 3 exercises (2 sets each)
E. *Biceps:* 2 exercises (3 sets each) or 3 exercises (2 sets each)

Day 3
Repeat Day 1, but vary the way you do the exercises (reps, speed, drop set) or pick different exercises.

Day 4
Repeat Day 2, but vary the way you do the exercises or pick different exercises.

If you're going to train four days per week with a more advanced workout style, follow this.

Day 1: Legs
A. *Quads:* 3-4 exercises (3-4 sets)
B. *Hamstrings:* 2 exercises (3 sets)
C. *Calves:* 2 exercises (3 sets)

Day 2: Chest and Triceps
Chest:
A. 2 presses (3 sets)
B. 1 fly (3 sets)
C. High-rep burnout press (1-2 sets only)

Triceps:
A. 3 exercises (2-3 sets): Incorporate drop sets and supersets.

Day 3: Back
A. 2-3 row exercises (3 sets)
B. 1-2 pulls (3 sets)

Day 4: Shoulders and Biceps
Shoulders:
A. 1 press exercise (3-4 sets)
B. 1 side lateral (2-3 sets)
C. 1 rear lateral (2-3 sets)
D. High-rep fatigue press (1 set only)
E. 1 shrug exercise (3 sets)

Biceps:
A. 3 exercises (2-3 sets): Incorporate drop sets and supersets.

The next week, follow the same schedule, but remember to change the style you're using and/or change up the exercises. You can also change the order in which you do the exercises, although first, you're going to want to do your power exercise most of the time and start with the larger muscles.

If you decide that you're going to really push yourself and train five or six days a week, I highly recommend training each muscle group only once a week. You can break up your days into single-muscle groups and increase your intensity a lot while slightly increasing your volume of sets. You can increase the amount of sets you do, but not by more than four total per exercise. You can increase your sets, but don't exceed four sets per exercise for power exercises and three sets for isolation exercises. If, for some reason, you feel you need to do more, work on increasing the intensity of your speed reps and supersets, not on increasing the volume of sets.

We have one more muscle group to cover. This is one of the most misunderstood muscles to train: the abdominals (ABS). I can't count the number of people who tell me they need to "do more abs" to flatten out their stomachs. Let's make this real clear right now: **You can do abs all day long or get the greatest set of abs in the world, but if you have body fat around your mid-section, no one is going to see them.**

Training any muscle does not reduce the fat in that area. I know ads and companies want to tell you otherwise, but they're flat-out lying to get you to buy their products. I've never had anyone come up to me and say, "My legs are so fat that I need to squat every day to get them smaller." They say the opposite, "I *don't* want to do legs hard because I don't want them to get bigger." It just doesn't work like that. Fat is fat and muscle is muscle. **Fat cannot turn into muscle and muscle cannot turn into fat!** Period!

Abdominal muscle will recover faster than other muscles, but I still don't believe in training them every day. From my experience, if you train your abs really hard, you will get the best results training them every third or fourth day. If you're not training them extremely hard, then you could train them every other day. So work out what's best for you and fit them into your training program. When you're training properly and following the rules of training, your abs are being worked constantly whether you notice it or not.

So how do you get washboard abs? Developing the abs through the proper training techniques will develop them, but the only way you're going to see them is by dropping down your level of body fat. That means eating clean and probably doing a lot of cardio training to help you burn off the body fat. Once you get to your desired body-fat level, it won't be as difficult to keep it there—and you'll have the abs you've been longing for.

Chapter 12

Changing Up Your Workout

This is an important principle to put in place from the very beginning. It's all too easy to find the exercises you like and do best, then do them the same way all the time. Like training using the wrong principles, you will get good results at first. After a while, two things will happen. First, it will become routine and you'll begin to go through the motions of training, but lose that laser focus you had at the start. Second, your muscle will adapt to the workout and the results will begin to diminish. Trust me, you'll have that favorite exercise and want to always start with that one to see your strength gains. There's nothing wrong with doing your favorite exercises, but change up how you do them. Personally, I try to do a different workout every time I go to the gym. This will help you stay focused and keep your muscles guessing. Once you've been training a while, many people hit "autopilot" on their programs. Same exercises, reps, speed and order equal results staying the same and getting stuck on plateaus.

Now, how do you change things up? It's easier than you think. It doesn't have to be anything dramatic. For an example, we'll take one of the simplest exercises: the incline machine bench press. Once you find the right seat and handle adjustments for your body, they don't change. You will go through the same plane of movement every time. So how can you change up this exercise? One way is just in the order you do it, whether it's first, last or somewhere in the middle. For our example, we'll look at changing it up by using different techniques while keeping to our four basic fundamental rules. For our example, we will assume that this person can perform an incline machine press for 20 reps with a weight of 150 lbs. (Keep in mind, the amount of weight is not your focus—it's the muscle and doing the reps properly). These rep numbers are just examples, not exact numbers, of where your reps may fall.

Day 1

	Pounds	Reps
Set No. 1:	170	16x

All sets done to fatigue, with an equal amount of rest.

| Set No. 2: | 140 | 16x |

Approximately 45 seconds

| Set No. 3: | 110 | 18x |
| Set No. 4: | 80 | 30x |

Day 2

| Set No. 1: | 130 | 25x |

All sets done to fatigue, with an equal amount of rest.

| Set No. 2: | 130 | 20x |

Approximately 30 seconds

| Set No. 3: | 130 | 16x |
| Set No. 4: | 130 | 12x |

Day 3

| Set No. 1: | 160 | 18x |

This is a drop set with no rest between sets.

Set No. 2:	130	15x
Set No. 3:	110	12x
Set No. 4:	70	20x

Day 4

| Set A, No. 1: | 170 | 15x |

Single drop set, no rest between first two sets.

| Set A, No. 2: | 110 | 18x |
| Set B, No. 1: | 150 | 14x |

Catch breath and repeat drop set with lighter weight.

| Set B, No. 2: | 90 | 20x |

Day 5

	Pounds	**Reps**
Set No. 1:	150	12x

Slow the speed count down to 5 seconds and return slowly.

| Set No. 2: | 120 | 10x |

Repeat this for the first three sets with an approximate 45-second rest.

| Set No. 3: | 90 | 10x |

When the third set is complete, rest only 10 seconds.

| Set No. 4: | 90 | 18x |

Perform the fourth set at a controlled, faster pace for more reps.

Day 6

| Set No. 1: | 150 | 14x |

Performed extra slowly for 5 seconds or more (10-second rest).

| Set No. 2: | 150 | 12x |

Performed slightly faster than normal (45-second rest).

| Set No. 3: | 110 | 12x |

Performed extra slowly for 5 seconds or more (10-second rest).

| Set No. 4: | 110 | 10x |

Performed slightly faster than normal (no rest).

| Set No. 5: | 80 | 25x |

Fast but controlled.

Day 7

| Set No. 1: | 120 | 30x |

Normal speed (20-second rest).

| Set No. 2: | 120 | 24x |

Normal speed (20-second rest).

| Set No. 3: | 120 | 16x |

Normal speed (no rest).

| Set No. 4: | 80 | 30x |

Fast but controlled.

There are more variations you can come up with, but there are seven different ways to do the same chest press machine. By keeping with any of those seven different styles, you can further change up the workout by supersetting the chest press with another chest exercise, i.e. cable flies, dumbbell press or flies, pec dec, or Smith press. When I choose to superset two exercises, I will almost always perform the power or heavier exercise first, then move to a lighter or more isolated exercise. When finishing with a lighter exercise, I usually pick a machine or cable exercise. On these exercises, I will also throw in half reps at the end, once I can no longer perform a proper full rep. This will help add to your strength and further fatigue the muscle.

All of the variations of this exercise can be transferred to all other exercises as well. With other exercises, you may also change hand or foot position, depending on the exercise. The options are almost endless. Be creative and challenge yourself and avoid doing the exact same thing every workout. Not only can you change the order of the exercises you do, but you can change and throw in different exercises.

Another way I like to change things up is one day I'll focus on a lower-reps range: 12-15 for upper and 15-20 for legs. The next day, I will focus on a higher-rep range: 20-plus for upper and 30-plus for legs. As your endurance improves, try lowering your rest time between sets and exercises. You'll have to lighten the weight, but this is a great change up if you have to get in a quick workout. You should be able to finish your workout 30-40 percent faster while fully fatiguing the muscle and getting a great pump and burn on them. In the beginning, I'd definitely preplan your workouts in order to try all these different styles and prevent getting stuck on one routine.

Once you've mastered reading your body and knowing all the exercises, you can go by how you feel that day. Listen to your body and train accordingly. Remember, a good workout isn't about going heavier than the last workout; it's about focusing on and training the muscle to its full capacity. When you're done, if you have a great muscle pump and think back and can say, "Wow, I couldn't have done another rep on any set that I did," then that's the type of workout that builds champions!

Now that I'm in my maintenance phase on training, sometimes my daily goal is to see how fast I can get in and out of the gym while still completely fatiguing the muscles I'm training. Keep in mind that fast never means compromising rules No. 2 and No. 3. I adjust my routine by time, supersets, drop sets and/or giant sets while reducing the weight and quickly resting the muscles to fatigue. When training this way, sometimes I feel like I could have done more, but after looking back at the session, I realize I couldn't have done another rep on any exercise I did. That's success, and it will keep improving your body.

Another way to mix up your training routine is by doing giant sets. As a general rule, you would do your heavier power exercise first, then a lighter power exercise, followed by an isolation exercise. There is no rest between these sets. Rest 1-2 minutes after completing each giant set. You could add on a fourth set to your giant set, but remember, no more than three rounds total. (When performed properly, that will be plenty and you'll be at full fatigue).

If you are not sure where your skill level and ability are, it's always better to start more slowly and with lighter weights. As you improve, you will begin to increase your intensity and your weight, as well as your number of sets and exercises. You can add more as you improve, keeping in mind it's the quality of each rep and set that counts.

It's a good idea to write out your workouts before you go to the gym. Know ahead of time what exercises, rep range and styles you're going to use. This will force you to keep mixing it up. Also, make a note of the amount of weight you're using for a particular style so you can later look back and see how far you've come. This will help keep you motivated and on track to hit all your goals.

Another thing to change up is your goals. I know you've already written them down, but as you begin to hit your short-term goals, you may think of other new, short-term goals to keep shooting for until you hit your medium-term goal. You may surprise yourself as to what you're able to accomplish, so keep adjusting your goals to push yourself and stay motivated. Never forget rule No. 1: Stay consistent and you will persevere. Your daily goal of "training days" is only achieved by getting to the gym. **Even a bad training session is better than no training session.**

One thing to *not* change: If at all possible, stick to your training days and times. Not only will this help keep you consistent, but your body adjusts to the time of day you train and you'll stay on track. Even if you don't feel like going or you're short on time, go! You'll be glad you did, and you'll probably get a better workout than you thought.

Chapter 13

What to Expect from Your Training

I've gone over this before, but it's so important, we'll touch on it again. **When you're training with your focus on the muscle and not on the weight, while using proper form, you're not going to be able to lift as much weight as you think, or could, if you were doing it improperly.** Your goals are to look and feel better, not to compete in a power-lifting competition. The muscle is going to be worked harder and you'll feel a more direct burn. It's normal for the muscle to feel extremely weak when you're done. Again, that's how you get the results you want. It's not that the muscle is weak; it's that you've completely fatigued it. Great job!

In the first few weeks, you will experience post-training muscle soreness. This is normal, even if it's sore to the touch. What happens is you actually get micro-tears in the muscle cell, and some of the intracellular fluid will leak out, putting pressure on the nerves, making the muscle very sore. After a few weeks of training, the muscle cells will adapt to your training and you won't have that type of soreness. Once you've adjusted to training, you should be able to feel that you trained your muscles, but they shouldn't be sore to the touch. You will be training harder and more intensely, but you won't have that type of soreness you did at first. You'll be surprised at how fast your muscles will adapt to your new training. If you continue to have that type of soreness, you're over-training and need to look at what you're doing and make some adjustments. Some people think being really sore means they got a good workout. Once your body has adjusted to this type of training, the only time you should be that sore is when you radically change something up. Then it's okay, as your muscle will adapt again and your body will keep improving. Sometimes after a very hard workout, I would think, I'm going to be sore tomorrow, only to find out the next day that I wasn't sore at all. I got the best workout I could, and my body was handling the intensity better. Also, sometimes I didn't think I had the best workout, and the next day I was sore because I had changed something up that my body wasn't used to.

You should also notice that you are getting a little stronger almost every week or that you can do more reps than before. Your strength will come up first, but it takes longer to see the changes in the muscle. It's an ongoing process. I highly recommend taking multiple pictures of different parts or angles of your body every 4-6 weeks so you can see your improvement. The improvements happen continuously, but at a slow rate. Since you see yourself everyday, it's hard for you to notice your improvements. That's where pictures and friends will help show you how much you've improved. I've had clients who didn't want any pictures taken, and they thought they hadn't improved at all until they saw a friend they hadn't seen in a while, and the friend asked them, "What are you doing? You look amazing!" Then they realize how far they've come.

Have fun with creating new workouts and make it exciting by seeing your body push new limits and hit new highs. It's work, but you can make it fun!

Chapter 14

The Exercises

With the knowledge you have on how to train and put a complete training program together, we can now turn our focus to the actual movements of each exercise you will be doing. We will cover the basic exercises for each muscle. You may not *do* every exercise we cover, but it's important to understand the theories and reasons behind each one. Knowing the basic exercises will help you transition to other, more complicated exercises. Your goals and skill level will determine what you choose to add in or take out. Also, **if you have an injury that a particular exercise exacerbates, don't do that exercise**. There are many alternative exercises to pick from. All of the basic exercises we cover should be available at almost any gym. Once you understand how the basic exercises are properly performed, while following my fundamental principles, you will be able to add in exercises and make adjustments to the same exercises for new ways to improve your body. Once you understand the four basic rules and see how the exercises are performed, you will be able to confidently walk into any gym—anywhere—and know exactly what to do. You will be on a direct mission to go in and complete a fantastic workout, which will put you on the path to achieving all your goals. From my experience, after you have read this book, you will know more than 90 percent of the people in the gym know. **Be confident in yourself and in your program, get it done and reach your goals!**

The following photos will show you the proper range of motion and plane of motion you need to follow to be successful. Pay close attention to the angles and positions of the body for each exercise. Once you master these movements, you will be on your way to a stronger and better you.

We will go though each muscle group one at a time. A special thank you to one of my fabulous trainers, Nell, and my 70-year-old client, Cynda (who proves that age is just a number), for helping me out with these exercise photos.

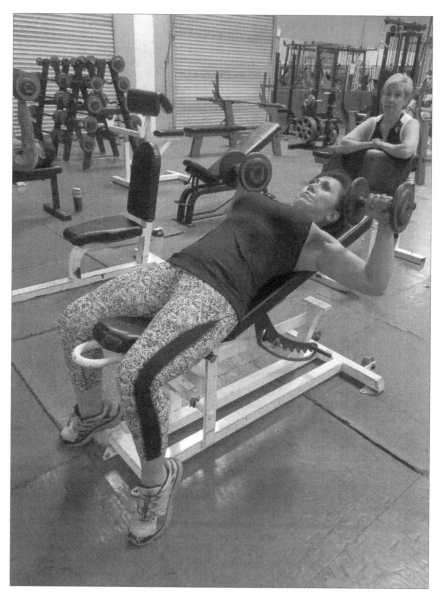

Incline Dumbbell Press

The bench should be at a low incline (15-30 degrees). Bring the weight down just past a 90-degree angle of the elbows.

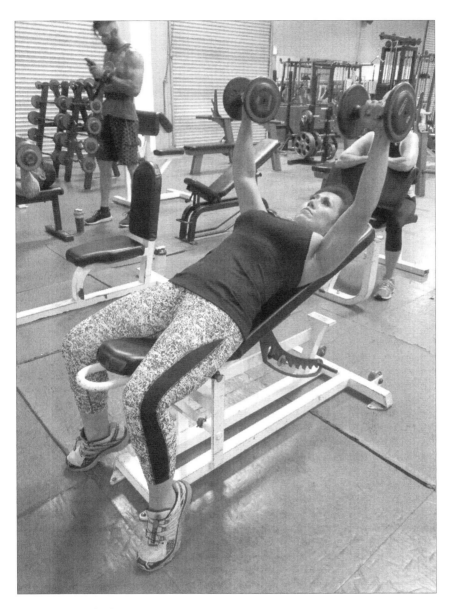

Incline Dumbbell Press

Push straight up without locking out. Avoid bringing the dumbbells together at the top, as doing so will take away from the chest and put extra stress on the shoulders and bicep tendon.

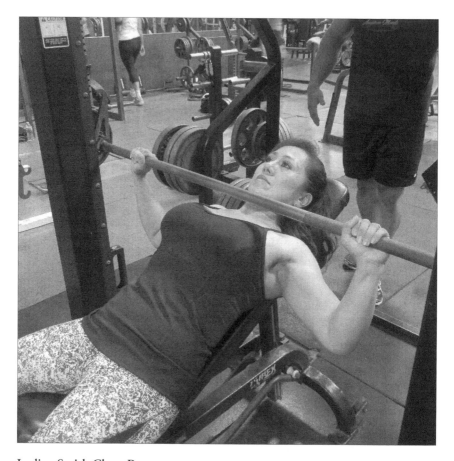

Incline Smith Chest Press

With a low incline, set the bench so the bar will come down at the top of your chest.

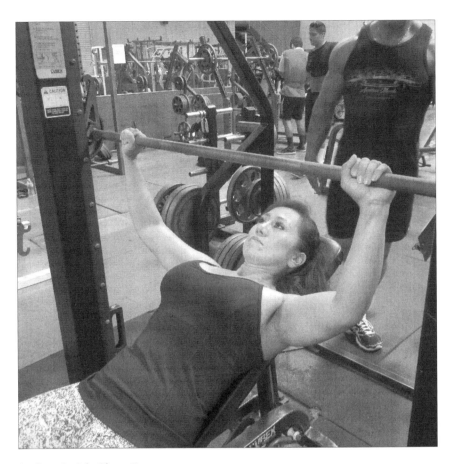

Incline Smith Chest Press

Keep your elbows slightly out as you go through the movement. Avoid locking out at the top.

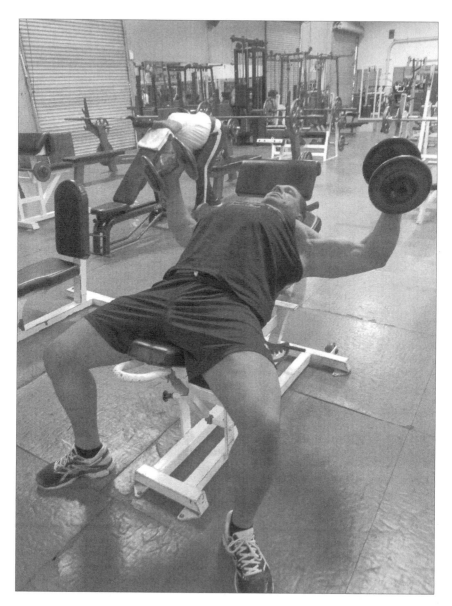

Dumbbell Incline Fly for Chest

Your elbows are bent at an approximate 140-degree angle (you will keep this same angle position throughout the entire range of motion). Keeping the elbows rotated slightly out, bring the weight down as far as possible without breaking your set angle (this will give you a full stretch—going any deeper takes the focus off the chest).

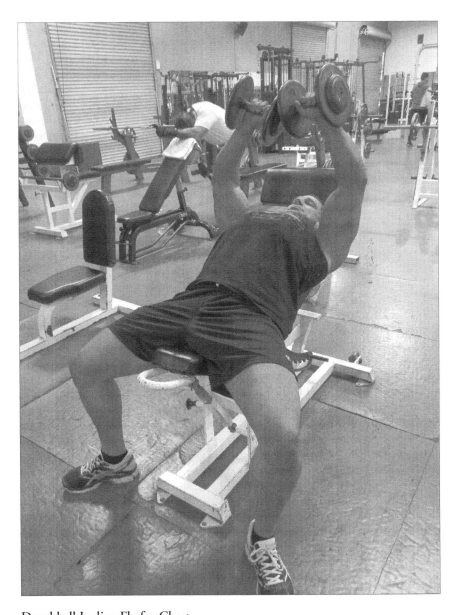

Dumbbell Incline Fly for Chest

As you get to the top, rotate the dumbbells together to get a better squeeze on the chest.

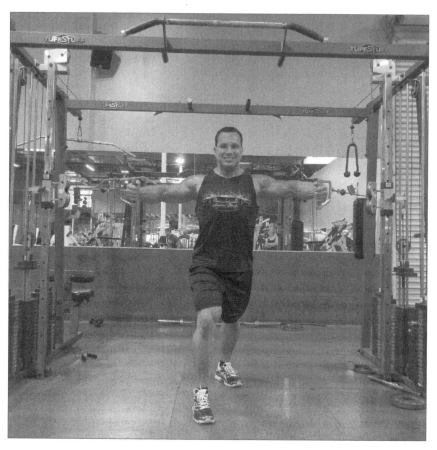

Cable Chest Fly

Your elbows are bent at an approximate 120-degree angle. Keep that same angle throughout the entire range of motion. Your elbows will be slightly rotated up and your arms should remain close to parallel to the floor throughout the movement.

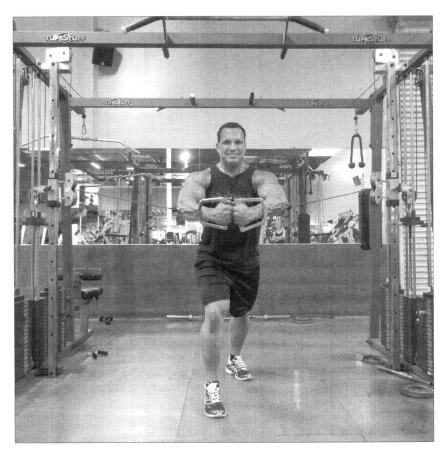

Cable Chest Fly

Get a full stretch without breaking your angle, and then get a hard squeeze of the chest as you bring your hands together.

*Elbows always stay slightly rotated up.

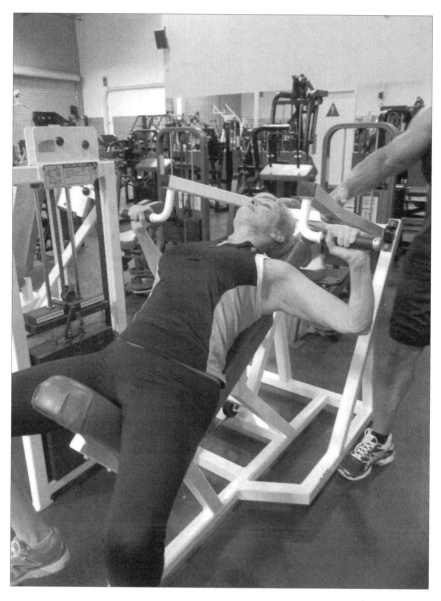

Incline Machine Press

Elbows are out and chest is up.

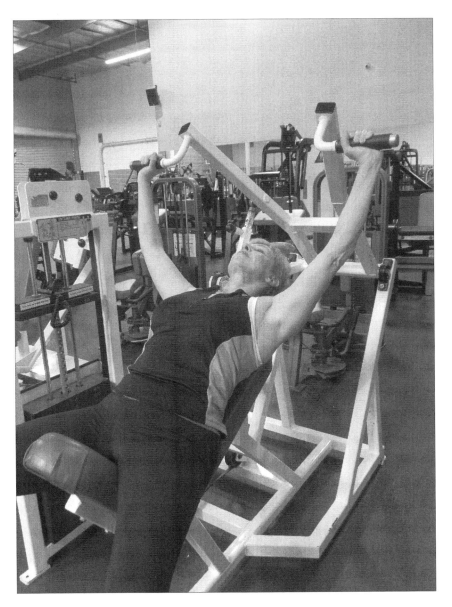

Incline Machine Press

Push up without locking the elbows, then come down smoothly with a good stretch and then go back up.

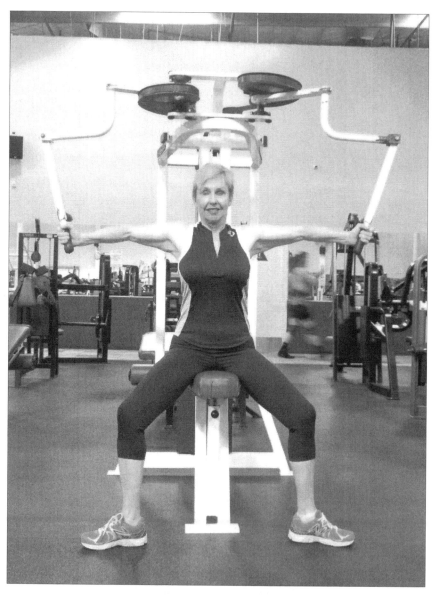

Pec Dec Fly

With your back straight and chest up, grab the handles, keeping your elbows bent and rotated up.

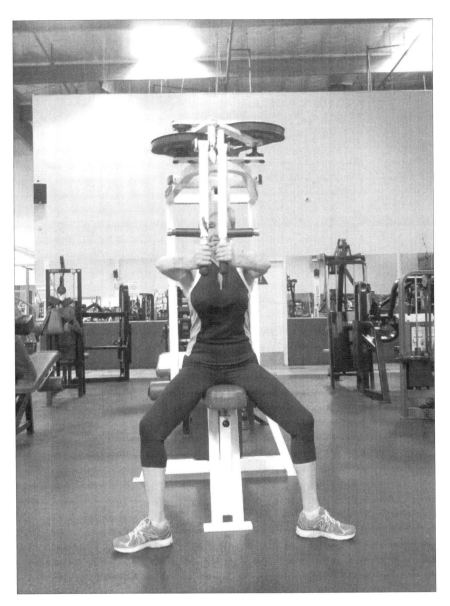

Pec Dec Fly

Bring your hands together, squeezing your chest at the top. Your arms should be parallel to the floor throughout the entire movement. As you come back with the weight, let your chest stretch without breaking your arm angle.

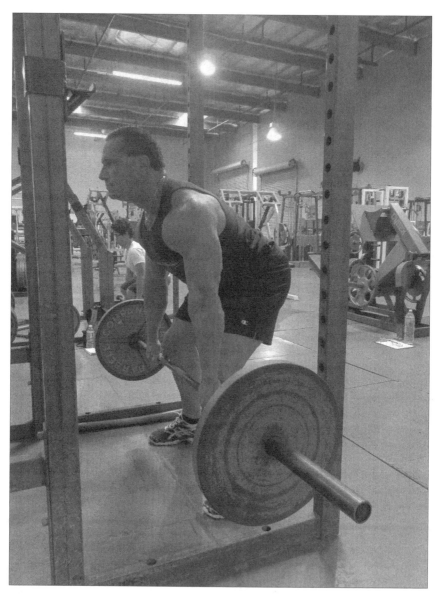

Free Bar Bent Rows

Bending over while keeping your back arched and your hips out, lower the bar down without losing the arch in your back.

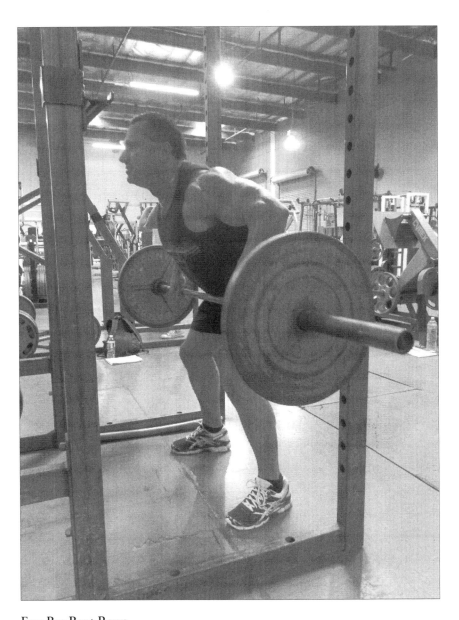

Free Bar Bent Rows

Pull up into your mid-section with the elbows out.

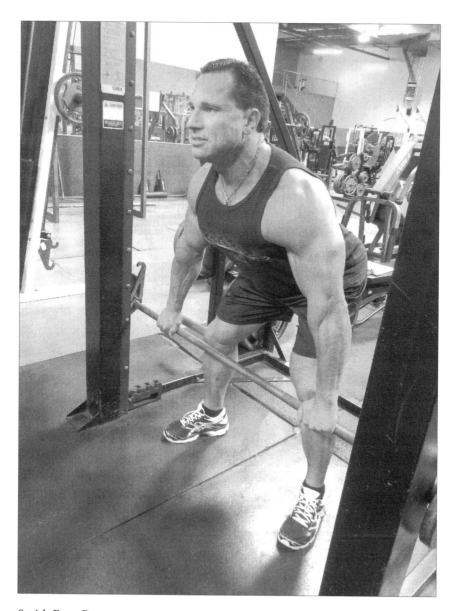

Smith Bent Rows

Your feet are shoulder-width apart or more. Bending over the bar with your hips out and your back arched, lower the weight (keep your back arched the entire time and don't let your shoulders roll forward).

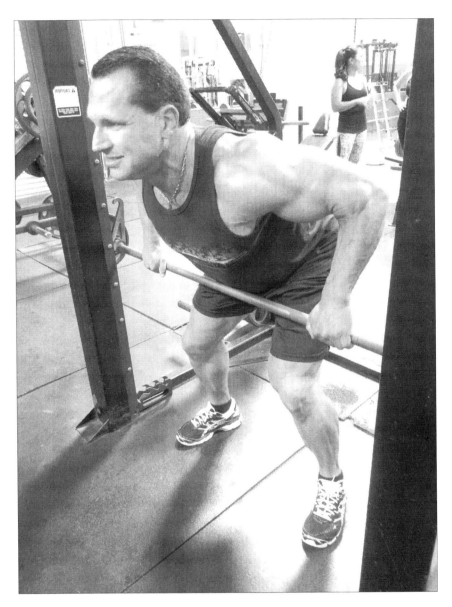

<u>Smith Bent Rows</u>

Pull the bar up into your mid-ab section while keeping your elbows slightly out and your back arched.

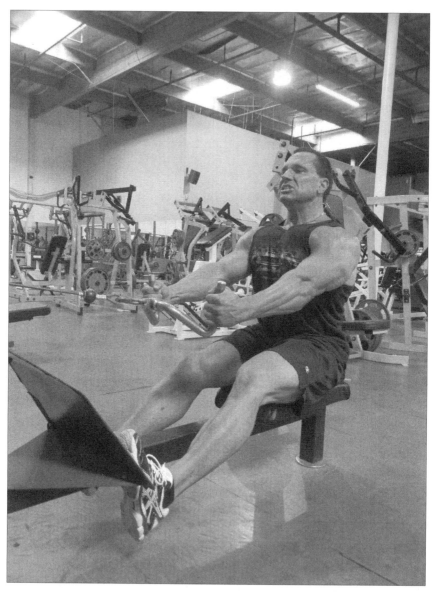

Seated Rows

Keeping your back arched and your chest up, pull the bar into your mid-section (feeling your back and shoulder blades squeezing together).

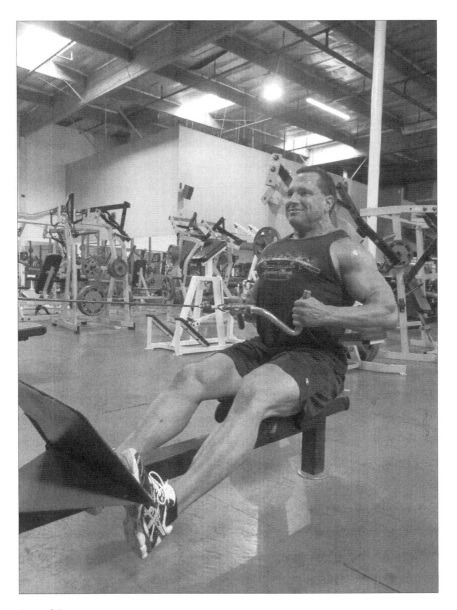

Seated Rows

You can let your back stretch at the bottom, but make sure to arch your back before pulling the weight back up again.

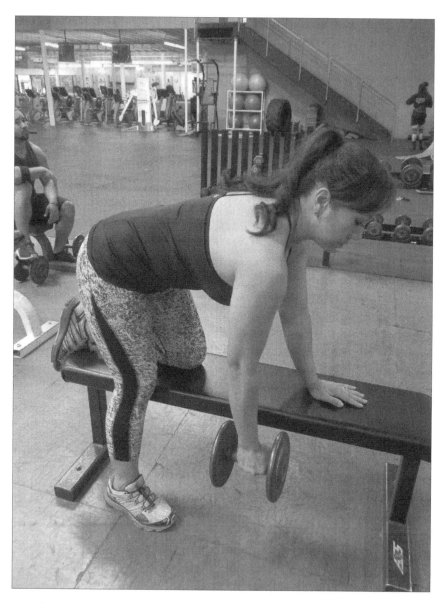

Dumbbell Rows

Start with your back straight and shoulders squared.

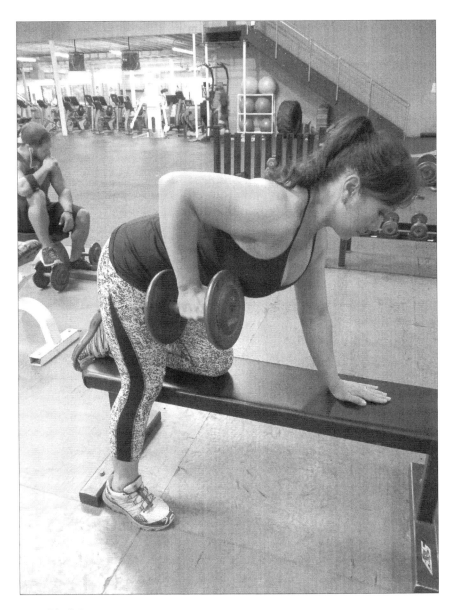

Dumbbell Rows

Pull up, keeping your back arched and the weight close to your body. As you lower the weight, you can let the back stretch, but make sure to keep your back straight.

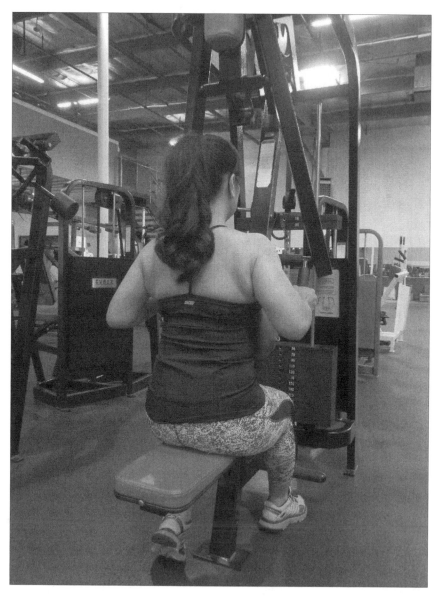

Machine Back Row

For balance, your feet can be in front of or behind you.

Arch your back and pull the handles as far back as possible while squeezing the middle of your back together.

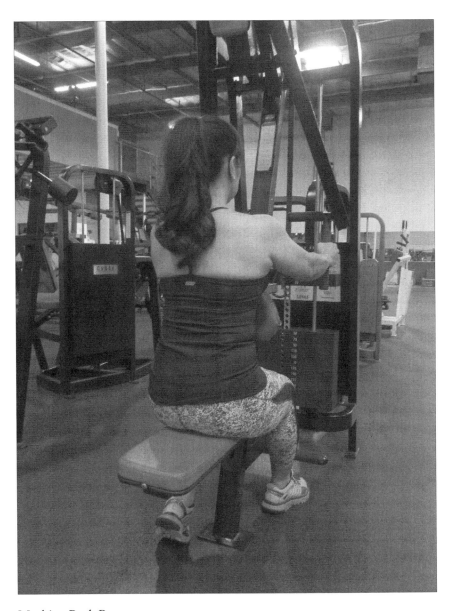

Machine Back Row

Return for a full stretch.

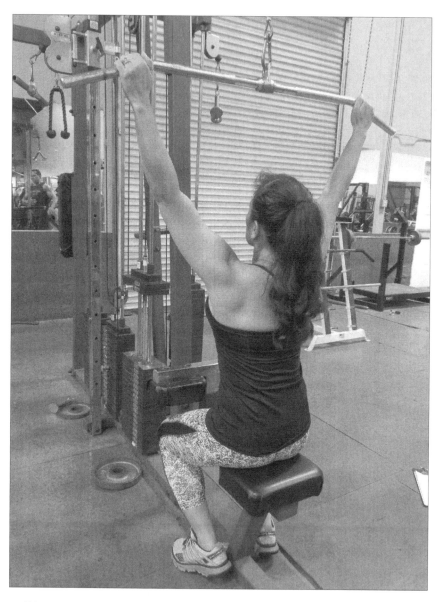

Pulldowns

Have your back arched and chest up.

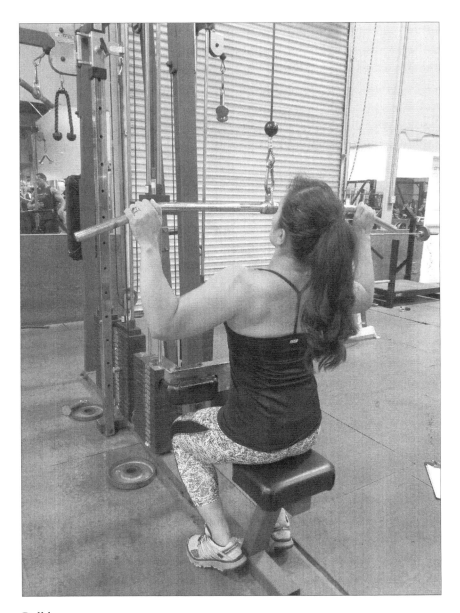

Pulldowns

With a wide grip, pull down with your elbows slightly out, bringing the bar to about chin level. Pulling down farther will take the pressure off the back, making the exercise less efficient.

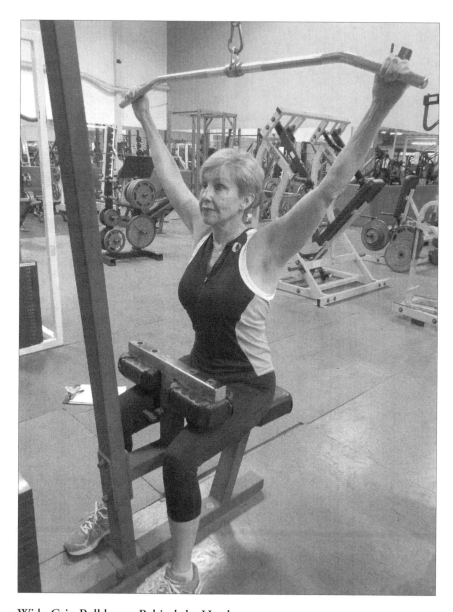

Wide-Grip Pulldowns Behind the Head

Start with a wide grip on the bar. Have your back arched and chest up.

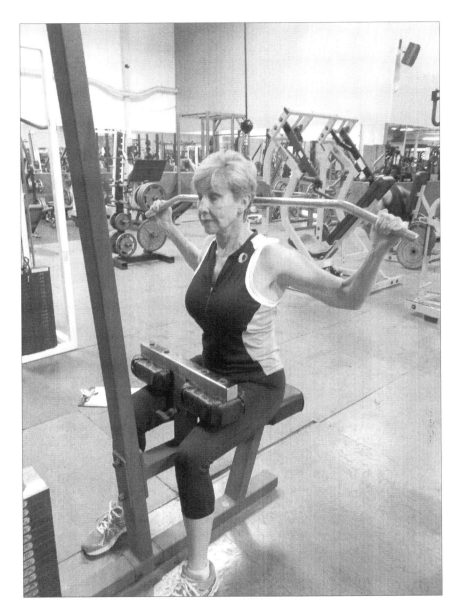

Wide-Grip Pulldowns Behind the Head

Leaning forward about 10 degrees, pull the bar down to the base of your head while keeping the elbows rotated out. Feel your shoulder blades come together at the bottom.

*Never pull the bar down past your head.

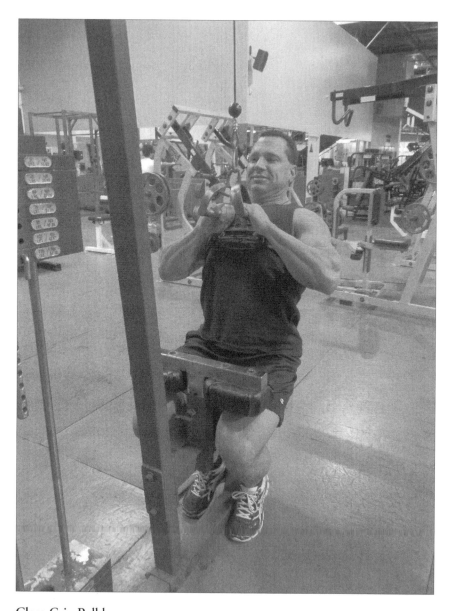

Close-Grip Pulldowns

Arching your back and keeping your chest up, pull the bar down to the top of your chest.

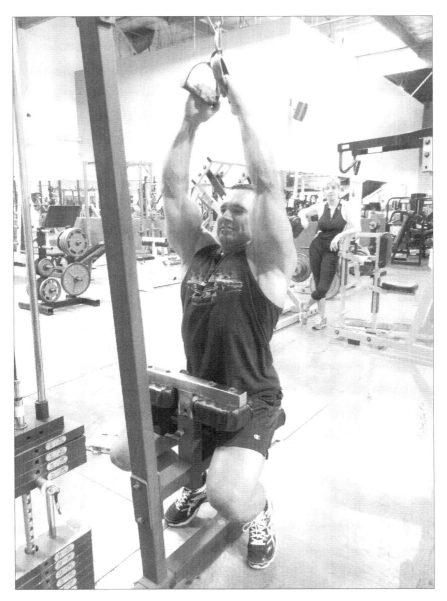

Close-Grip Pulldowns

As you come up, you can let your back stretch at the top, then arch again and pull down.

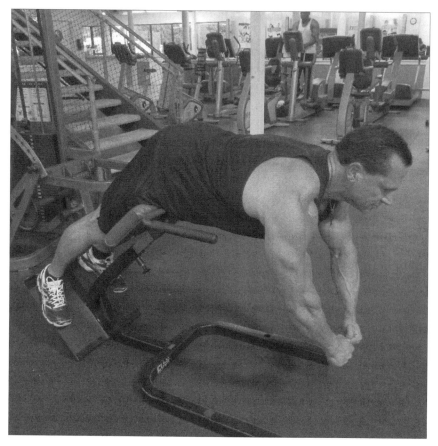

Hyper Extensions

Adjust the seat to have your knees just below the pad. Arching your back with your chest up, lower your upper body down as far as possible without losing the arch in your back.

Hyper Extensions

Once you've hit that spot, return to the top. Be careful to not over-extend at the top. While returning up, bring your elbows up to get an extra squeeze at the top of your back.

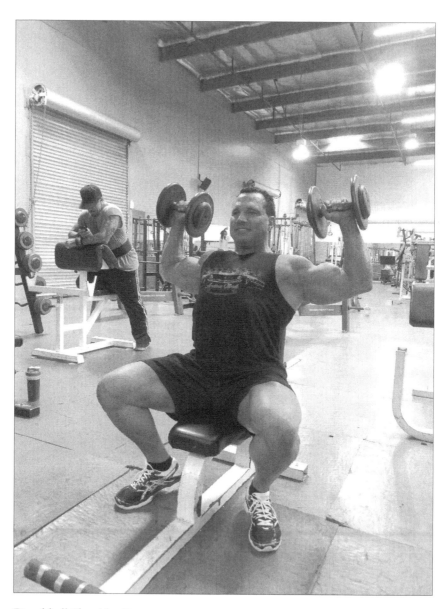

Dumbbell Shoulder Press

Have your elbows at 90 degrees or slightly less (80-85 degrees). Bring the dumbbells down just below a 90-degree angle (don't go deeper in the bottom).

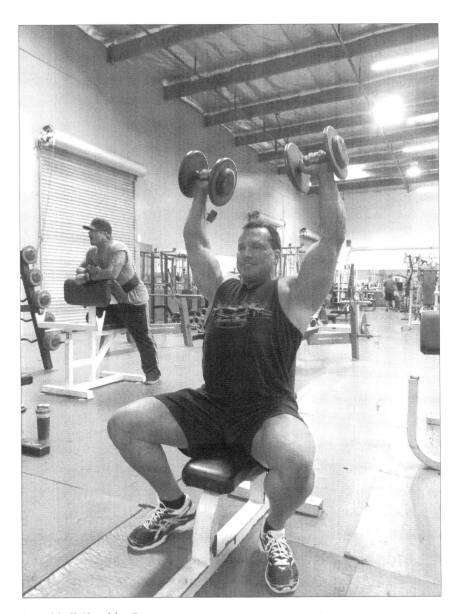

Dumbbell Shoulder Press

Push straight up without locking out the elbows. It is better to NOT bring the dumbbells together at the top. By avoiding this, you will keep more tension on the shoulders.

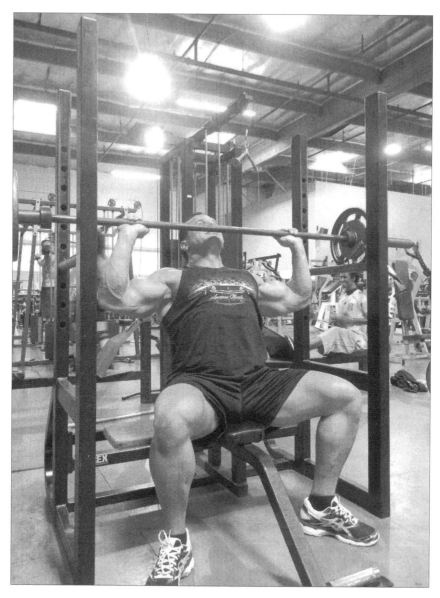

Free Bar Shoulder Press in Front

Using a shoulder-width grip or slightly less, slightly lean your head back and lower the bar to about chin level while keeping your elbows slightly out. Push up without locking the elbows.

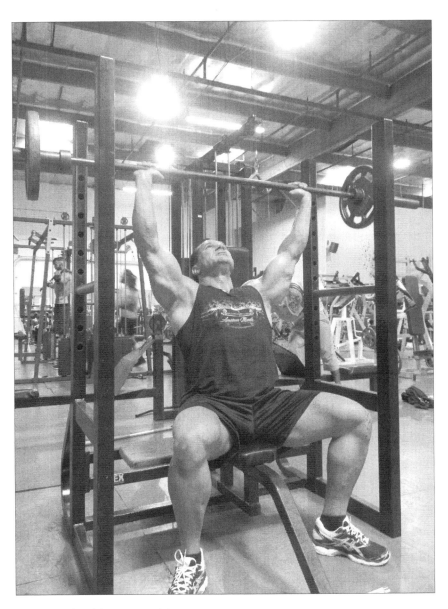

Free Bar Shoulder Press in Front

Push up without locking the elbows.

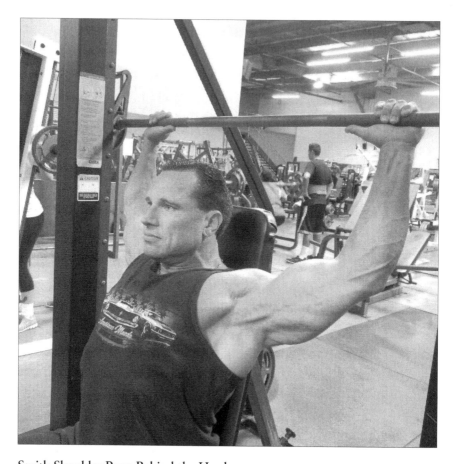

Smith Shoulder Press Behind the Head

Your elbows are at a 90-degree angle or slightly less when the bar is at the bottom of the exercise.

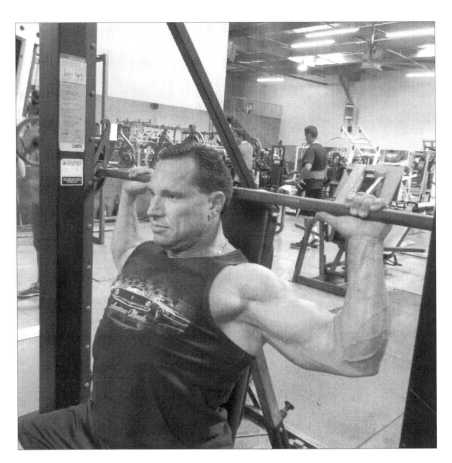

Smith Shoulder Press Behind the Head

Only bring the bar down to the base of your head or just beyond the 90-degree angle at the bottom (if you drop the bar down to your neck, you risk a shoulder or bicep injury).

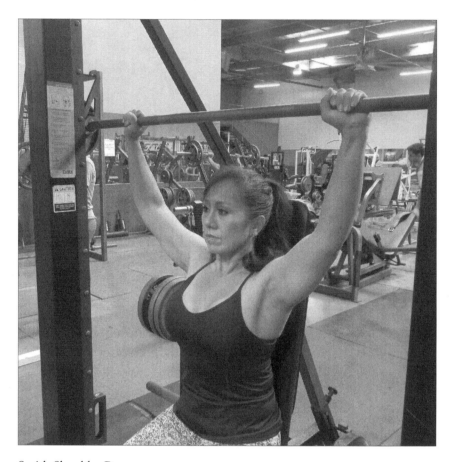

Smith Shoulder Press

Position the bench so the bar will come down just in front of your head.

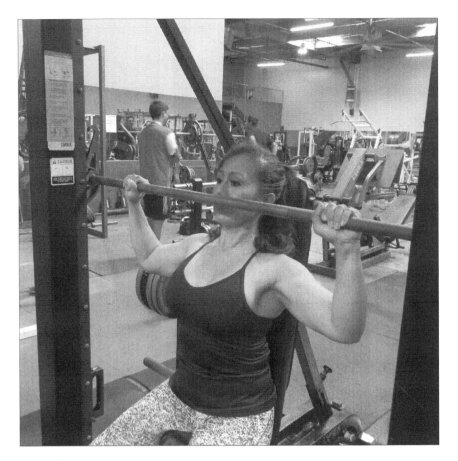

Smith Shoulder Press

With a shoulder-width grip, lower the bar down to your chin while keeping your elbows slightly out. Push up short of locking the elbows.

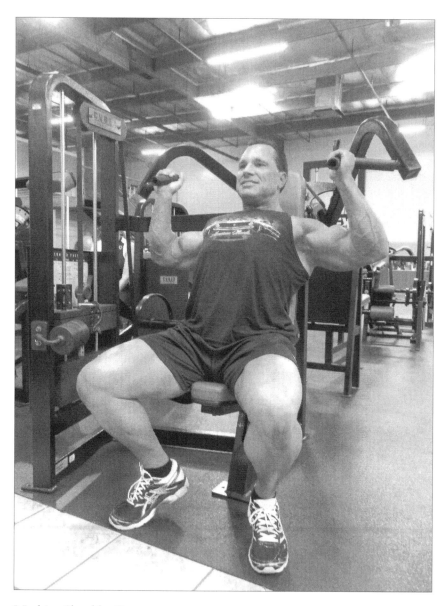

Machine Shoulder Press

Take a shoulder-width grip, keep your elbows rotated slightly out, and lower the bar down just below parallel.

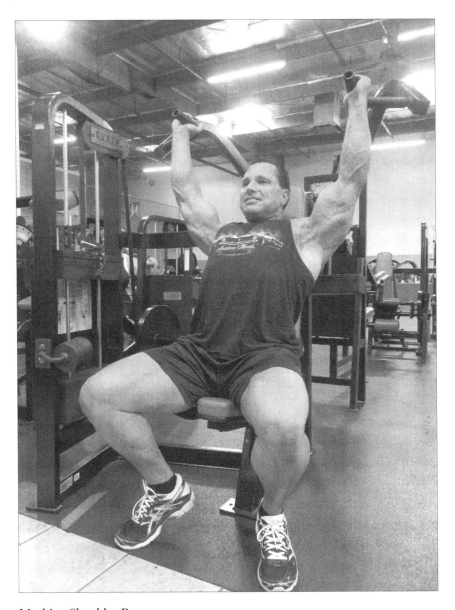

Machine Shoulder Press

Push up without locking out the elbows.

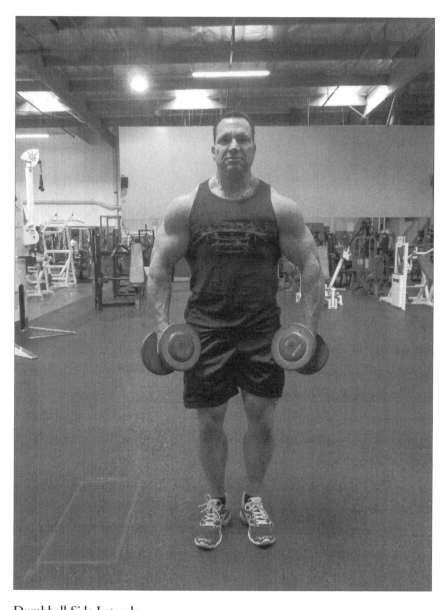

Dumbbell Side Laterals

Starting with the dumbbells at your side, have your elbows slightly bent.

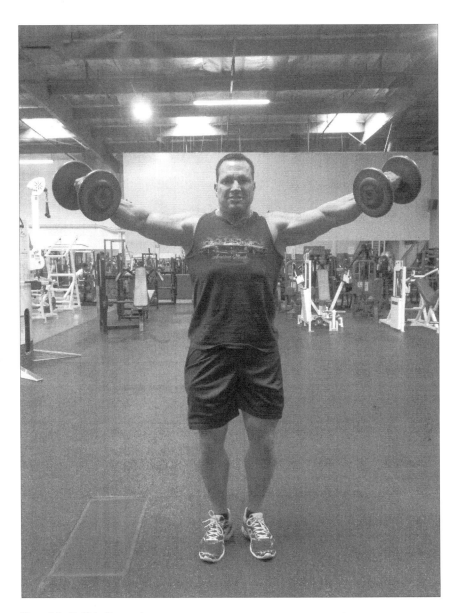

Dumbbell Side Laterals

Lift the dumbbells straight out to your side while keeping the same bend in your elbows. Keep the elbows rotated slightly out and up. Lift your arms until they go just past being parallel with the floor. Return to the bottom and repeat without using momentum to go back up.

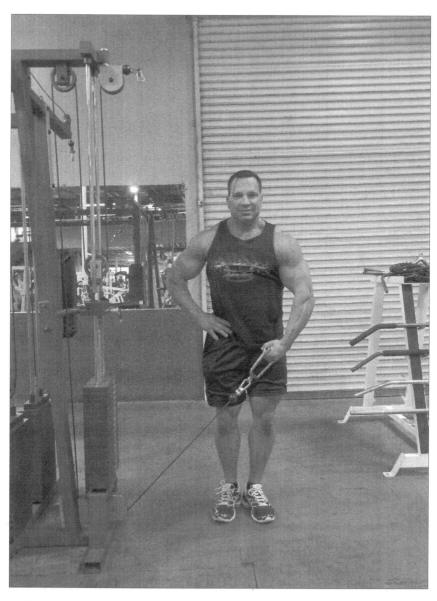

Cable Side Laterals

Have your shoulders and hips squared and put your other hand on your hip for balance and to help keep your body straight.

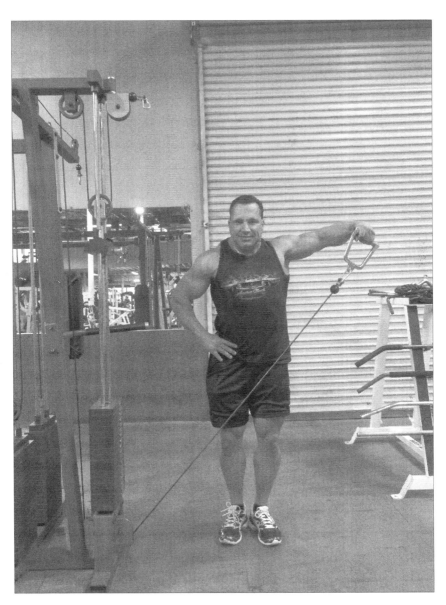

Cable Side Laterals

Pull straight out to the side, keeping your elbow rotated slightly up. Pull out so your arm goes up just past parallel. Return slowly and avoid using any momentum coming out of the bottom of the exercise.

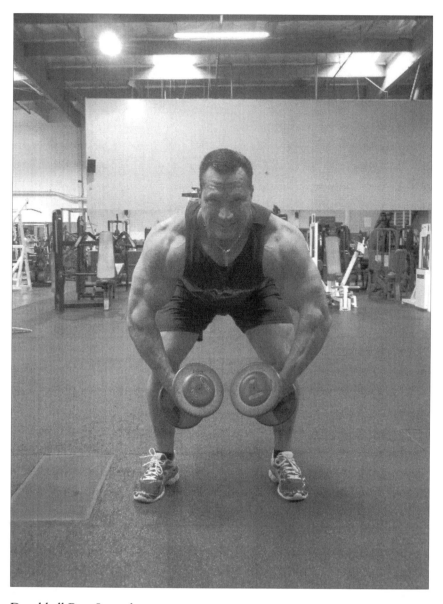

Dumbbell Rear Laterals

Bend over with your back arched, hips out and elbows bent.

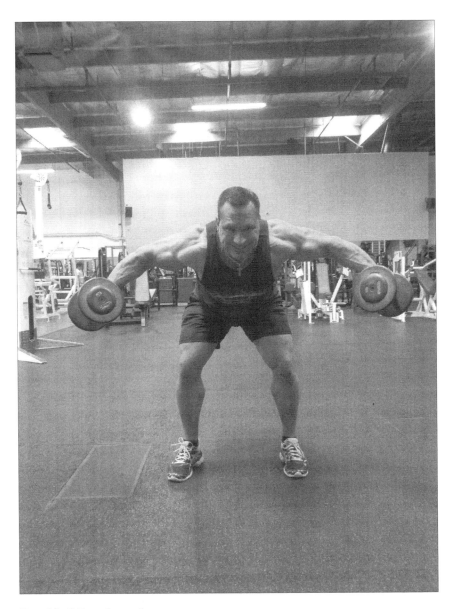

Dumbbell Rear Laterals

Pull the weight straight out from your body (not back behind your body). Squeeze your shoulder blades together at the top.

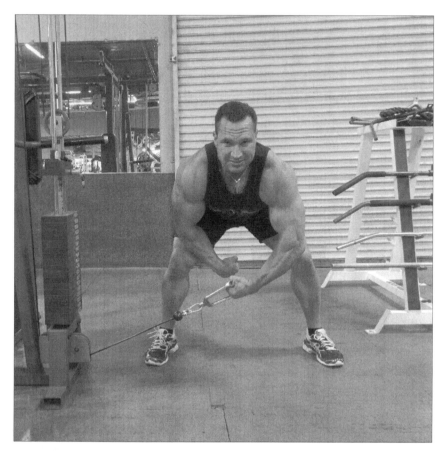

Cable Rear Laterals

With shoulders and hips squared, lean over, putting one elbow against your knee for balance.

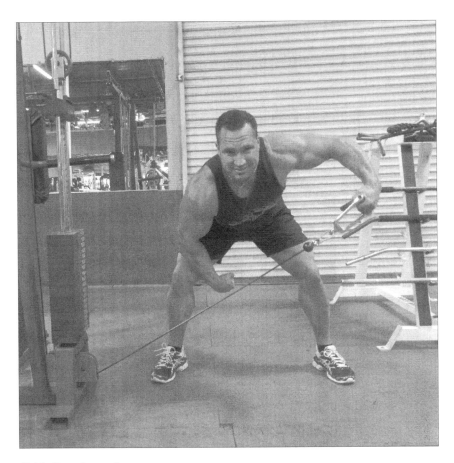

Cable Rear Laterals

With your other arm bent, pull straight out, leading with your elbow. Pull up without losing your arm angle.

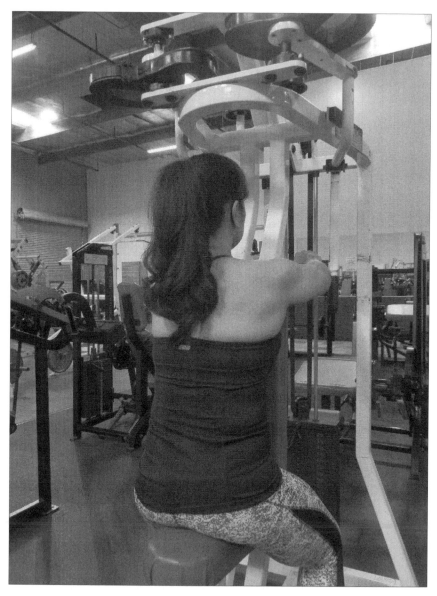

Rear Delts on the Pec Dec

Face the machine with your arms parallel to the floor and elbows bent and slightly up.

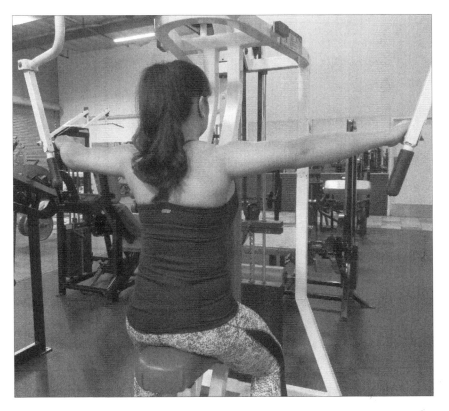

Rear Delts on the Pec Dec

Pull back while squeezing your shoulder blades and return with the same motion.

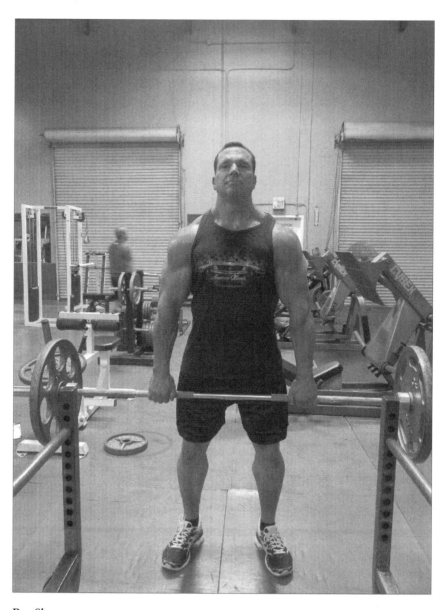

Bar Shrugs

Take a shoulder-width grip, keeping your back and head straight.

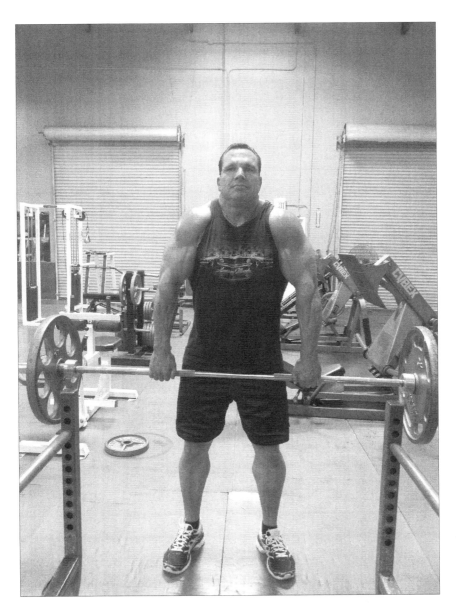

Bar Shrugs

Lift with your shoulders while keeping your arms straight. Come up as high as possible without bending your elbows, then lower and repeat.

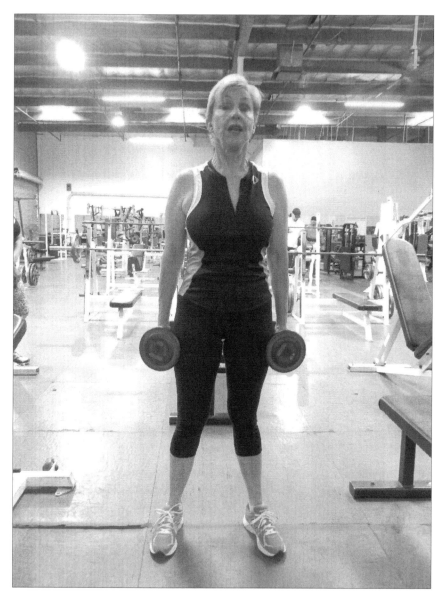

Dumbbell Shrugs

Same as barbell shrugs. You can change the position of the dumbbell from rear to side to front to change up the exercise.

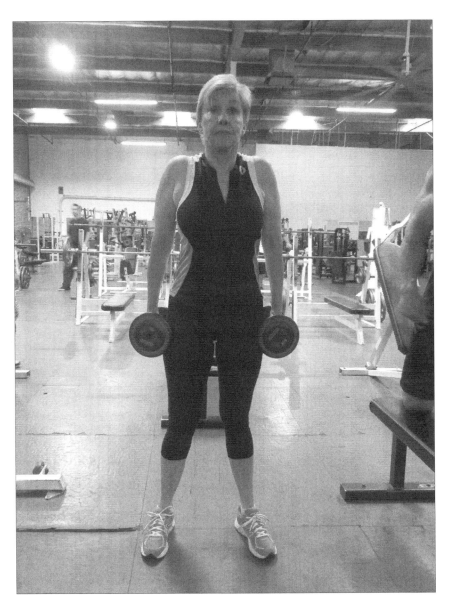

Dumbbell Shrugs

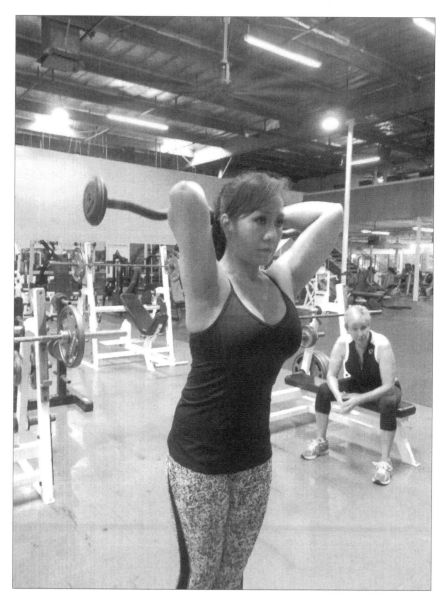

Triceps Extension Behind the Head

Using a close hand grip, let the bar go behind your head as far as possible while trying to keep your elbows in.

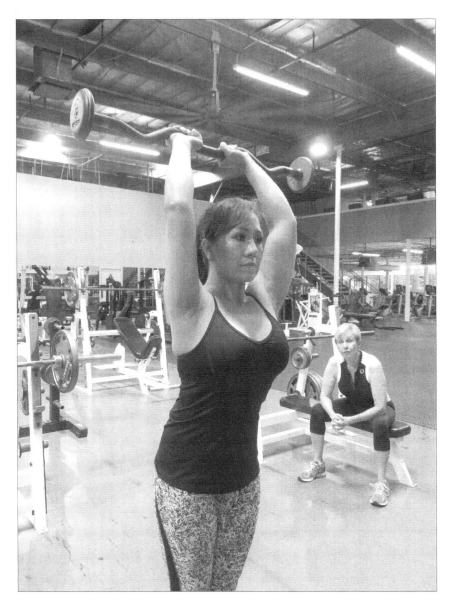

Triceps Extension Behind the Head

From the bottom of the stretch, push up while keeping the bar behind your head. Squeeze your triceps at the top of the movement.

*Avoid bringing the bar over your head, as this takes the pressure off the triceps.
*This exercise can also be done with a dumbbell or the rope from a cable machine.

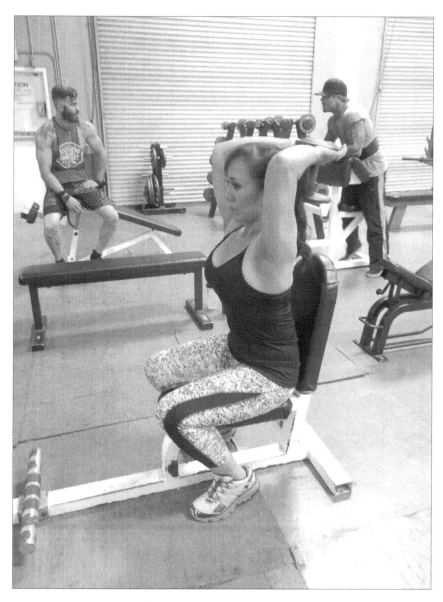

Triceps Extension Behind the Head

Using a close hand grip, let the bar go behind your head as far a possible while trying to keep your elbows in.

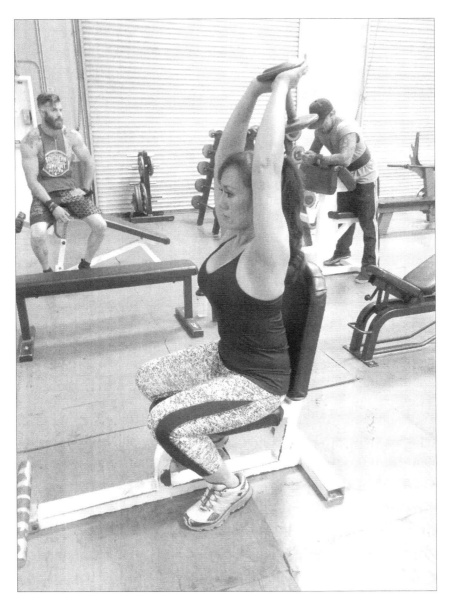

Triceps Extension Behind the Head

From the bottom of the stretch, push up while keeping the bar behind your head. Squeeze your triceps at the top of the movement.

*Avoid bringing the bar over your head, as this takes the pressure off the triceps.
*This exercise can also be done with a dumbbell or the rope from a cable machine.

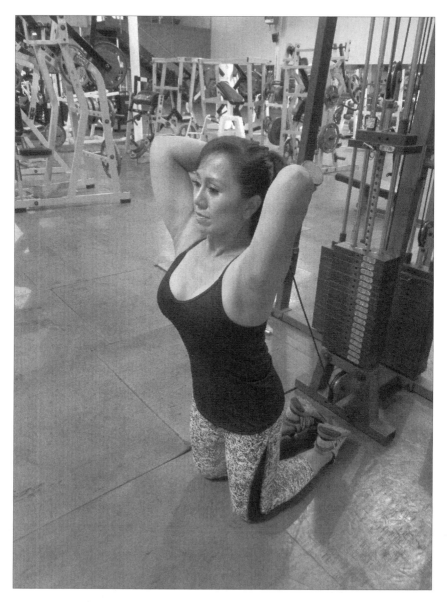

Triceps Extension Behind the Head

Using a close hand grip, let the bar go behind your head as far a possible while trying to keep your elbows in.

Triceps Extension Behind the Head

*From the bottom of the stretch, push up while keeping the bar behind your head.
Squeeze your triceps at the top of the movement.*

*Avoid bringing the bar over your head, as this takes the pressure off the triceps.
*This exercise can also be done with a dumbbell or the rope from a cable machine.

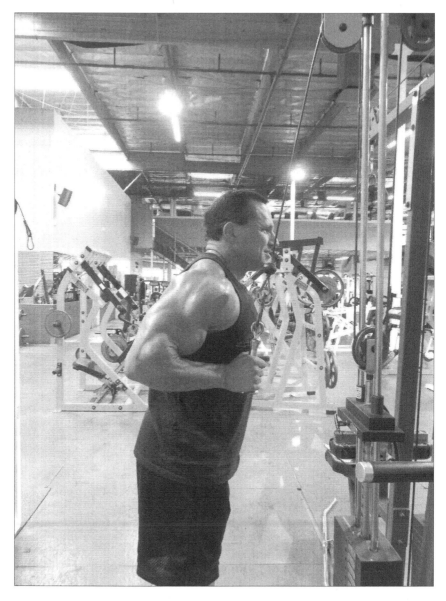

Single-Tricep Extension
Keep your shoulders squared and body forward.

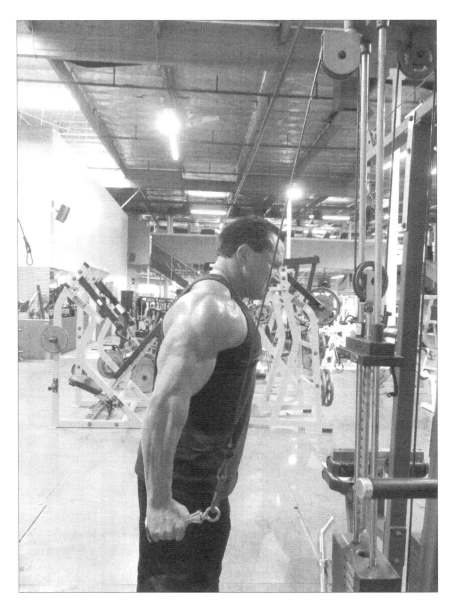

Single-Tricep Extension

Keeping your elbow back as far as possible, push straight down, squeezing your triceps at the bottom, then return the handle up, keeping your elbow back and in close to your body.

*Don't let your elbow come forward at the top.

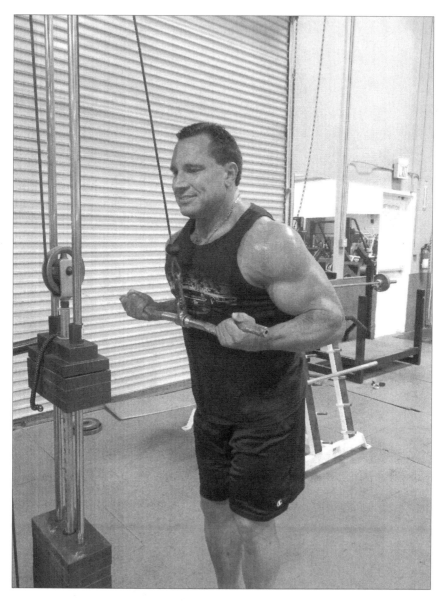

<u>Reverse-Tricep Pushdowns</u>

Grab the bar with an underhand grip.

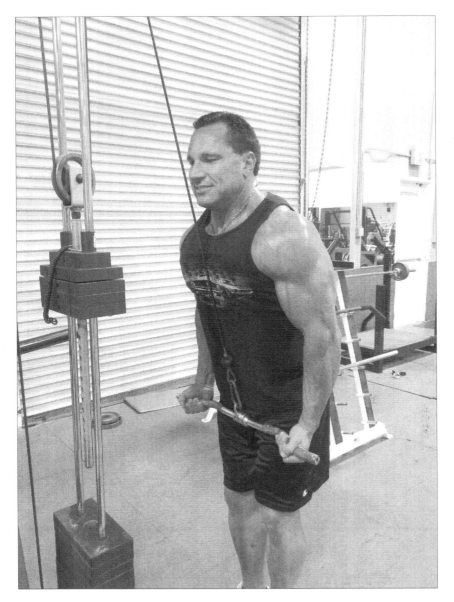

Reverse-Tricep Pushdowns

Keeping your elbows back and close to your side, pull the bar down (keeping the bar as close to your body as possible). Squeeze your triceps at the bottom, then return the bar up, keeping it as close to your body as possible again. Don't let your elbows come forward at the top (keep them back).

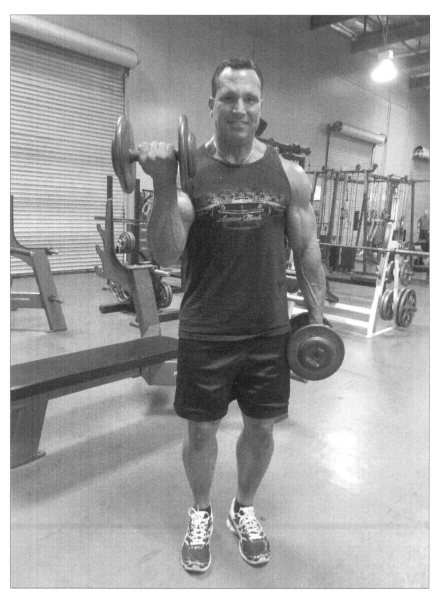

Alternating Dumbbell Curls

Twist one dumbbell out and curl slightly out and up, flexing the bicep at the top.

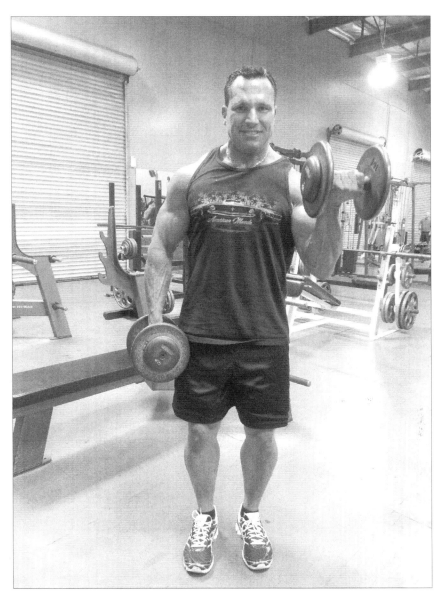

Alternating Dumbbell Curls

Lower the weight down, then repeat the same motion with the other arm.

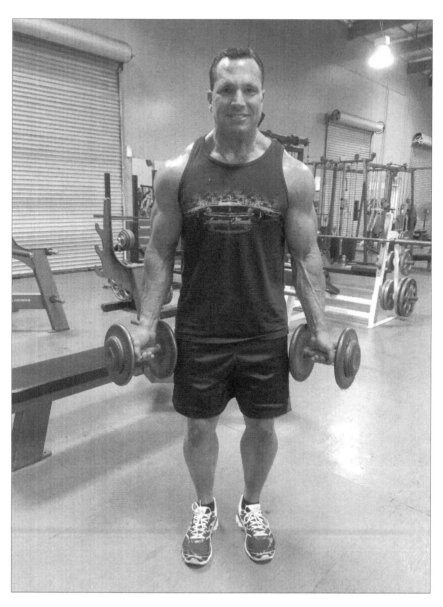

Double Dumbbell Curls

Twist the dumbbells out and curl up, keeping your elbows in close to your side. Bring the weight down and let it stretch at the bottom and repeat.

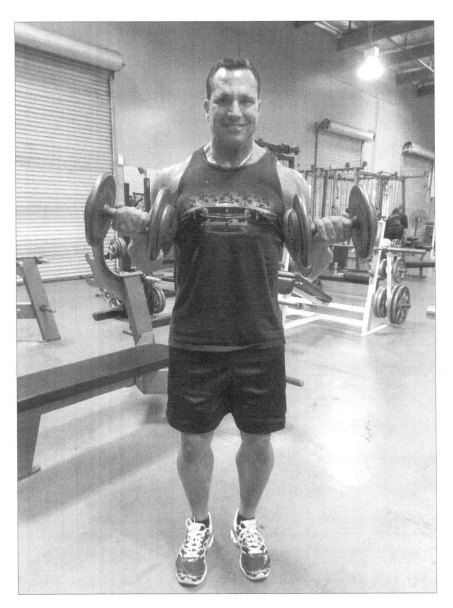

Double Dumbbell Curls

Always keep your elbows in close to your body, but you may move them forward or back on different sets to change the exercise.

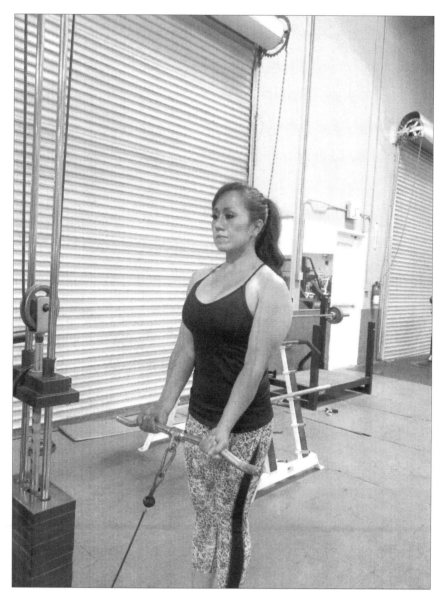

Bar Curl

This is performed the same way as the rope curl, but is done with heavier weight, as it is a power movement. You can also change the angles on this to hit different parts of the bicep.

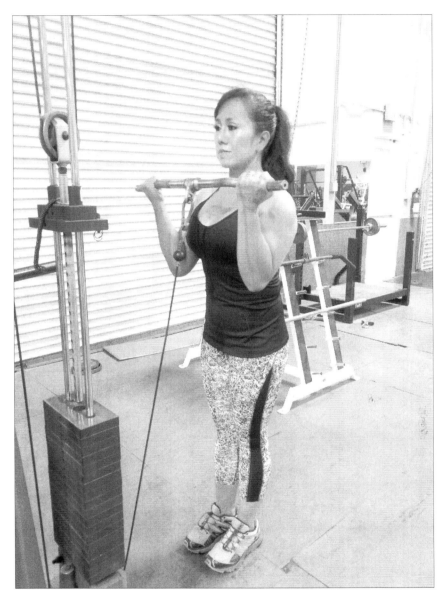

Bar Curl

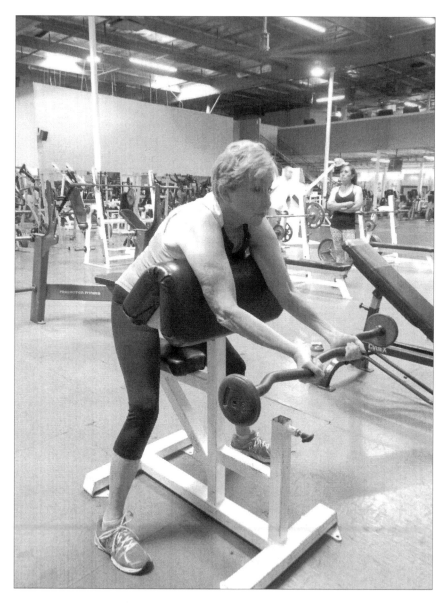

E-Z Bar Preacher Curls

Have the bench completely under your arms and slowly lower the bar down.

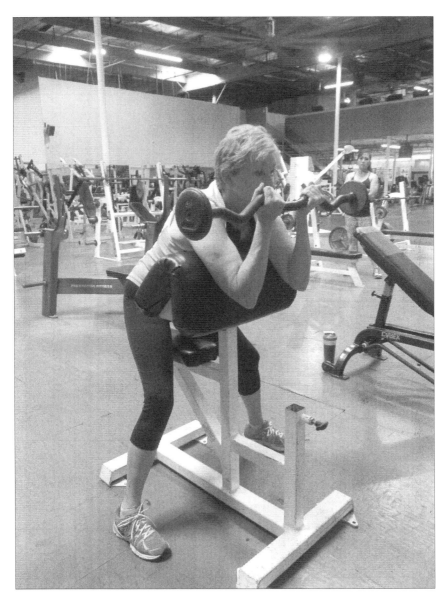

E-Z Bar Preacher Curls

With no bounce or momentum, squeeze the biceps as you come up and flex the biceps hard at the top. Elbows stay in close for the entire movement

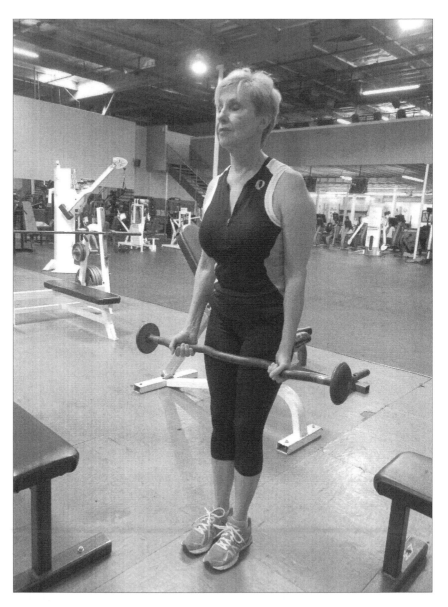

E-Z Bar Curl

Same form as the other curls. With this exercise, you can change up hand position from close to wide and also change the angle at which you bring up the bar.

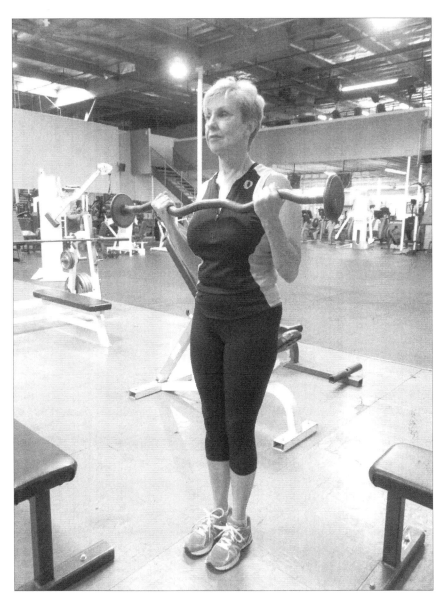

E-Z Bar Curl

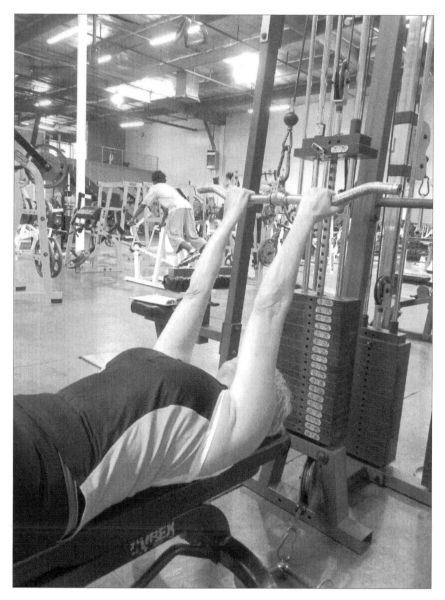

Lying Cable Curl

Lying on a flat bench, under the cable machine, grab the bar with a close grip.

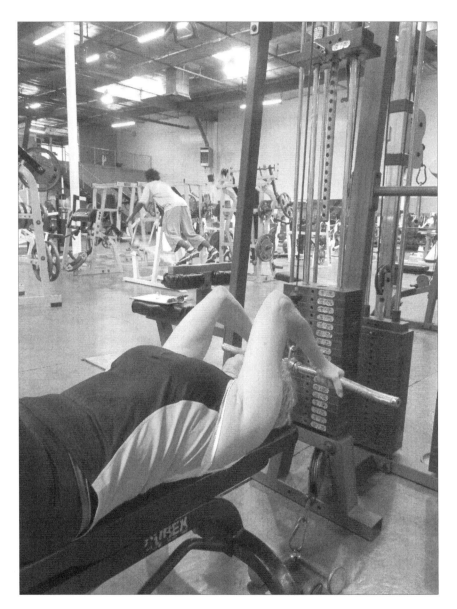

Lying Cable Curl

Pull the bar down behind your head, flexing the biceps at the bottom. On this exercise, you can change positions and hand grips to vary the exercise.

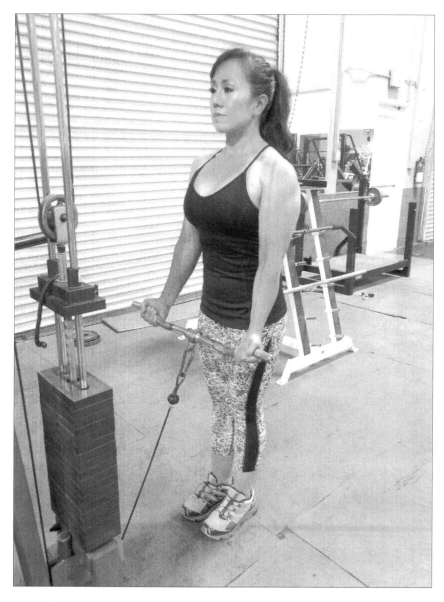

Cable Curl

Curl up and out with a hard squeeze on the bicep at the top. Return curling slowly out of the bottom with no swing and keeping the back straight.

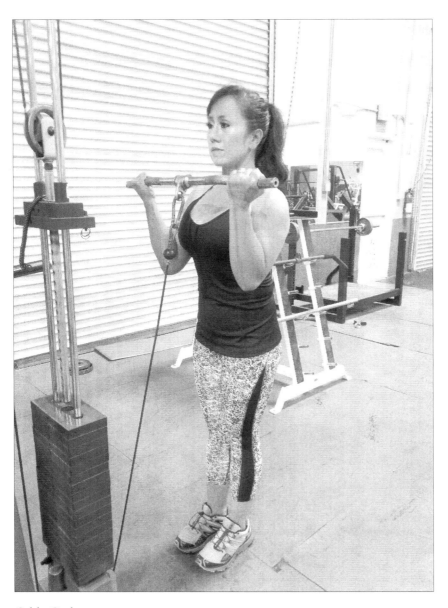

Cable Curl

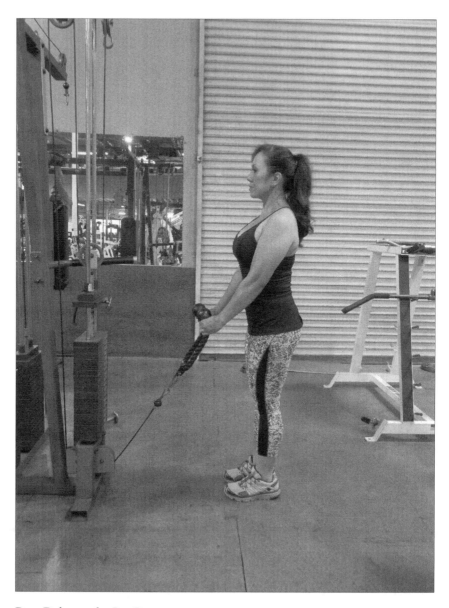

Rear Delts on the Pec Dec

Face the machine with your arms parallel to the floor and elbows bent and slightly up.

Rear Delts on the Pec Dec

Pull back while squeezing your shoulder blades and return with the same motion.

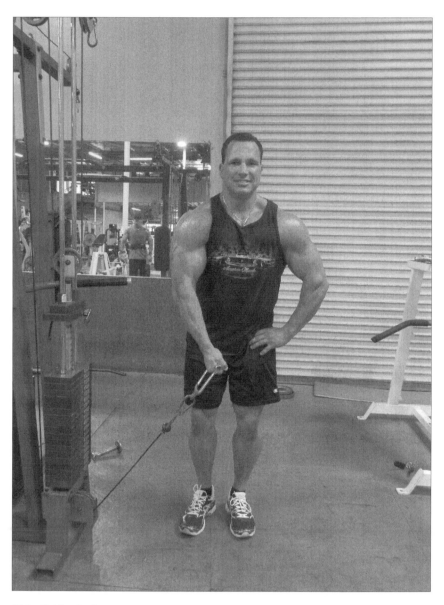

Side Cable Curl

Stand to the side with your shoulders squared.

Side Cable Curl

Curl up, keeping the upper part of your arm straight. Squeeze at the top and lower your hand slowly to the bottom.

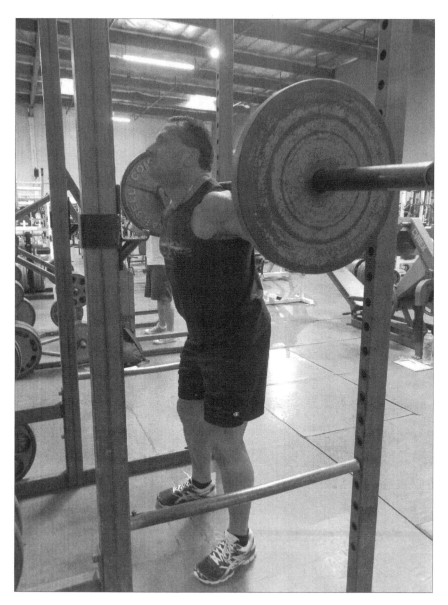

Free Bar Squat

The bar should be resting on the top of your shoulders (not on your neck). Feet are shoulder-width apart, with the toes pointed slightly out.

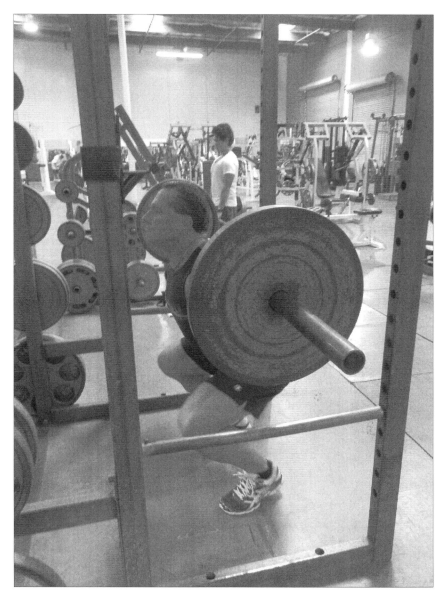

Free Bar Squat

Keeping your back arched and your head up, squat down (avoid leaning too far forward with your back). Then push up, stopping short of locking the knees out, and repeat.

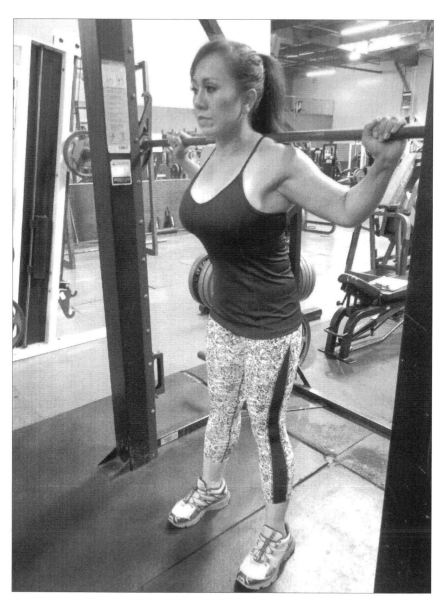

Smith Squat

Same position as the squat. Have the bar on the top of your shoulders.

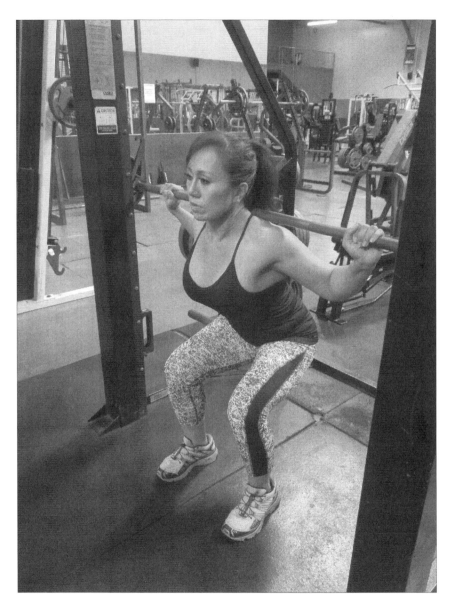

Smith Squat

As you squat down, your hips will go back and your shoulders will push back against the bar. Come down as far as possible, making sure to not bounce at the bottom, and return short of locking out the knees.

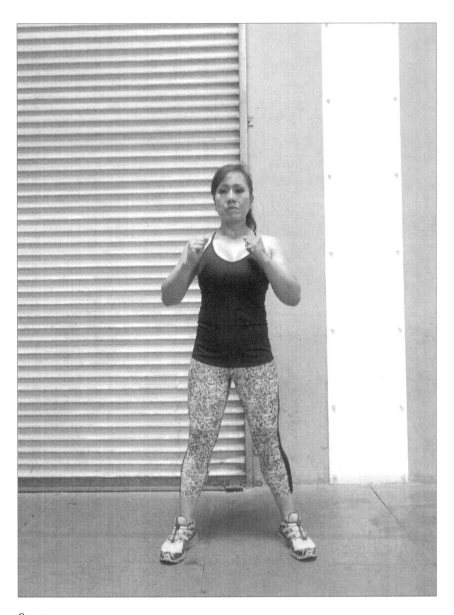

Squat

Stand with your legs shoulder-width apart and toes pointed slightly out. Keep your back straight and your head up.

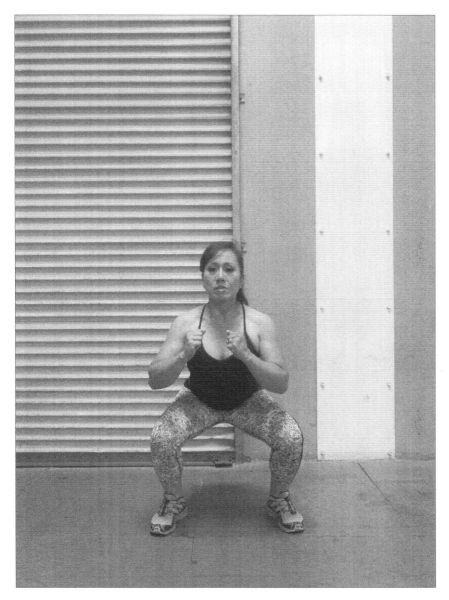

Squat

Squat straight down to a 90-degree angle and push up short of locking out.

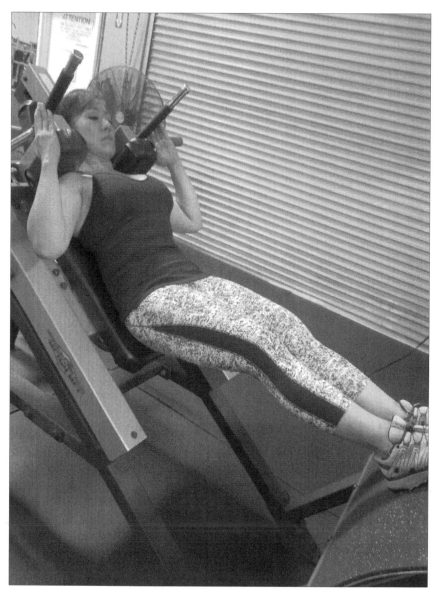

Hack Squat

The weight will rest on your shoulders. Keep your back and hips flat against the pad.

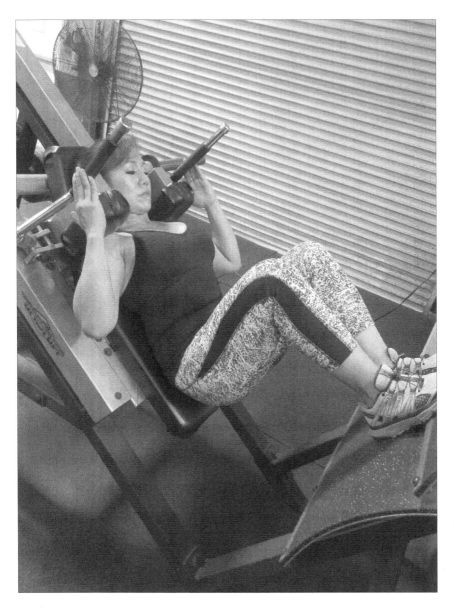

Hack Squat

Come all the way down, keeping your legs close together.

*You can change foot position to hit the legs differently.

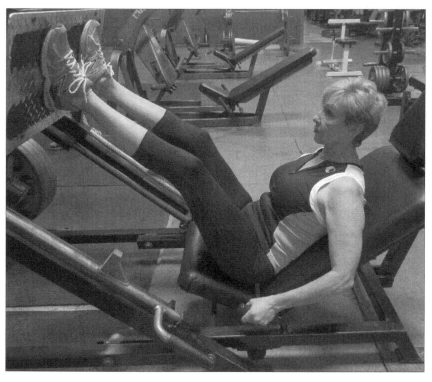

Leg Press

Start with your feet approximately shoulder-width apart and toes pointed out.

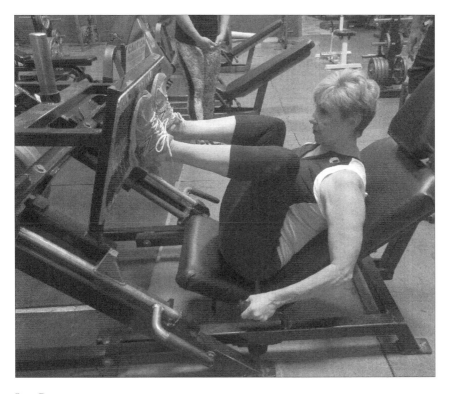

Leg Press

Lower the weight down and stretch as far as possible. Push back up without locking out the knees.

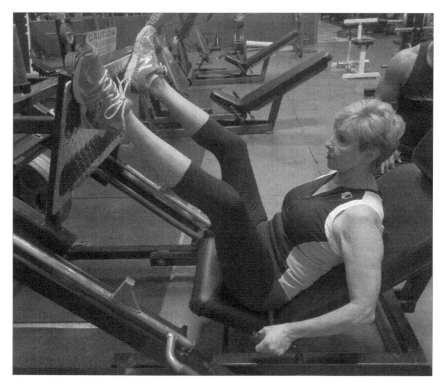

High, Wide-Leg Press

Your feet will be up high, wide and pointed out.

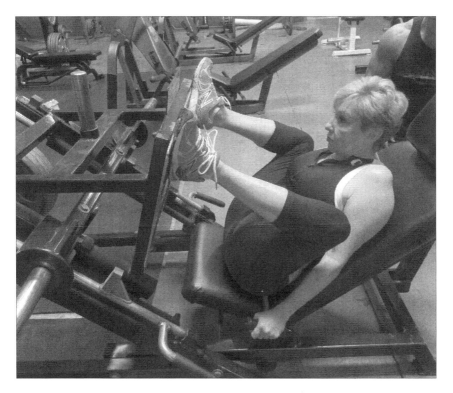

High, Wide-Leg Press

Let your knees go out as you come down. Get a deep stretch and push up through your heels to avoid locking out. This will help hit glutes, hamstrings, inner thigh and quads.

*When getting a full stretch, your hip will roll up some, which is okay. Just keep the weight controlled.

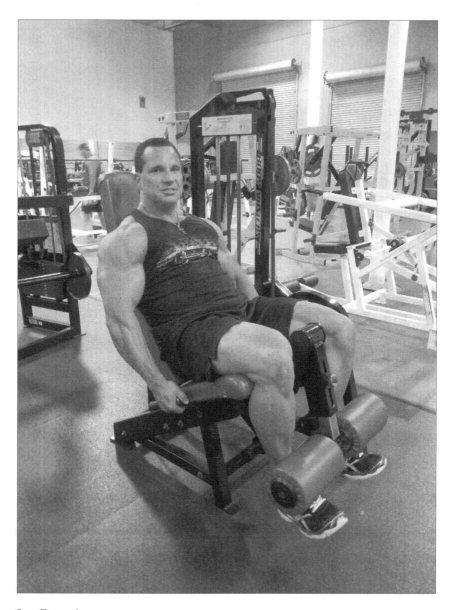

Leg Extensions

Adjust the seat so your knees are at the end of it.

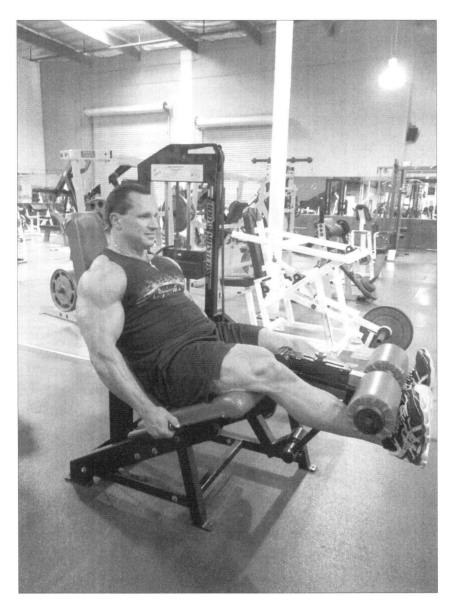

Leg Extensions

Slightly point your toes out and extend up, short of locking out the knees. Flex your legs at the top and lower the weight to the bottom, then, without resting at the bottom, return up.

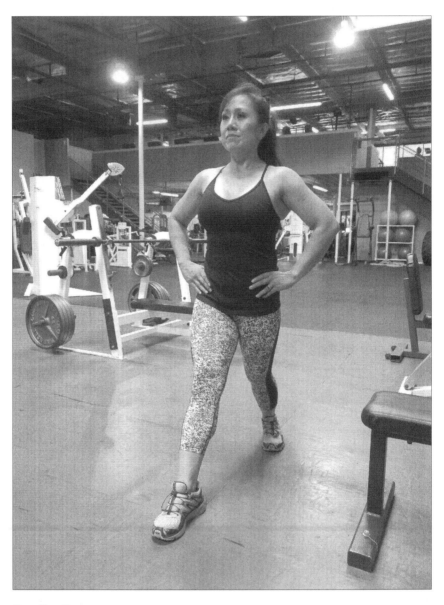

Standing Lunge

Have one foot in front and one in back and keep your back straight and head up.

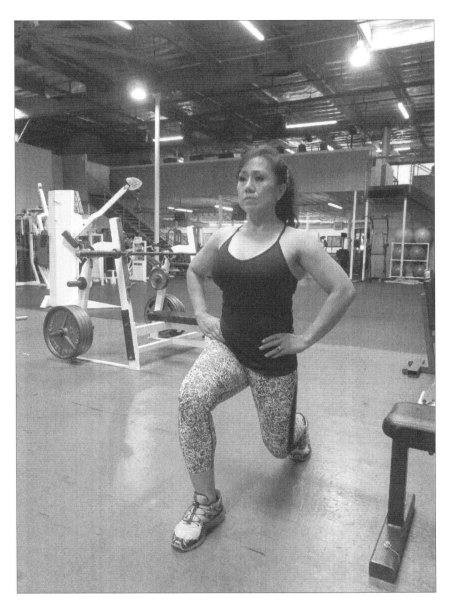

Standing Lunge

Bend the front leg and slowly come down without letting your knee go out over your front foot. Once you hit a 90-degree angle, push off your front foot and come up short of locking the knee out. In the beginning, you may want to hold onto a bar to help with balance and strength until you can do the exercise without assistance.

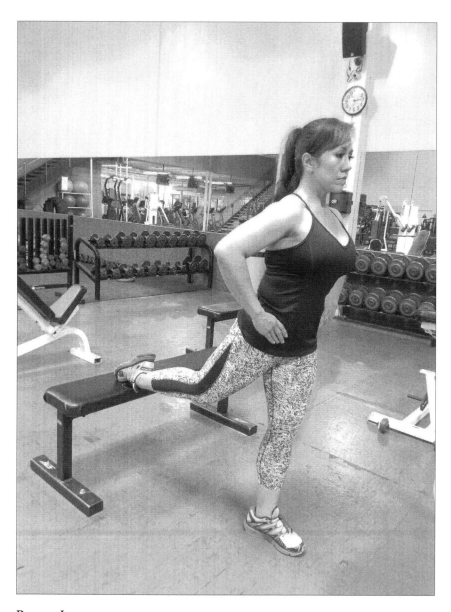

Reverse Lunge

Have your back foot on a bench with your front foot out. Back and hips are straight.

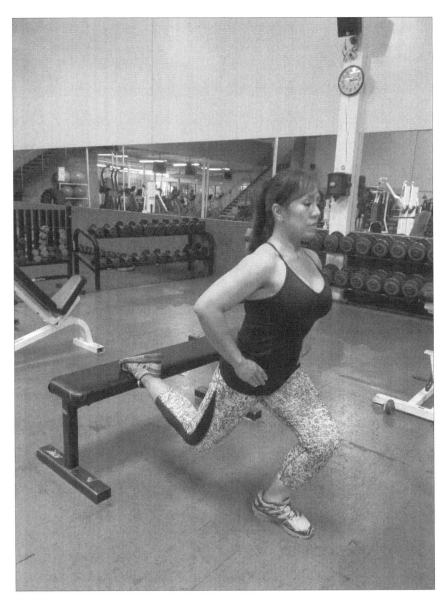

Reverse Lunge

Come down until your front leg hits a 90-degree angle (your knee doesn't go over your foot). Then, pushing off your front foot, return up short of locking out. Again, beginners may want to hold on to something solid for balance.

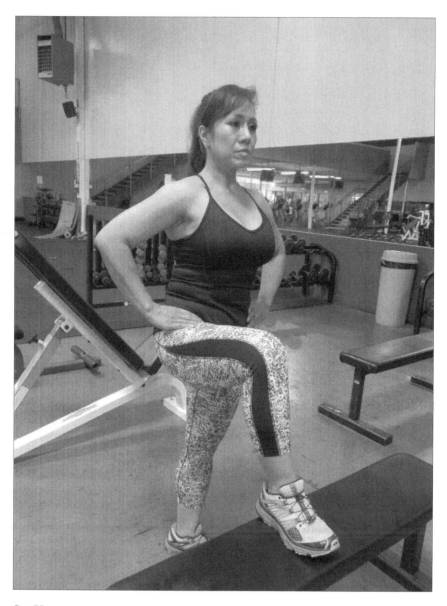

Set-Ups

Put one foot on the bench with the knee at a 90-degree angle.

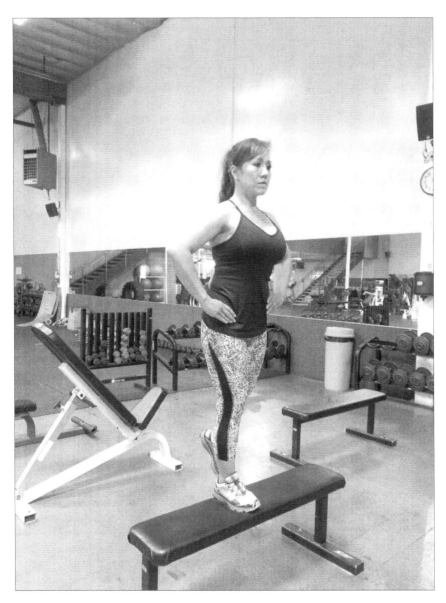

Set-Ups

Push off that foot, coming up just short of locking the knee to keep the tension on the leg. Do the same leg until failure then switch legs.

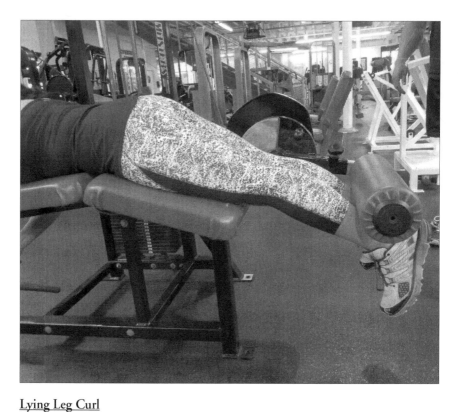

Lying Leg Curl

Position your body so your knees are just off the bench and the leg pad is above your ankles. Toes are pointed slightly out.

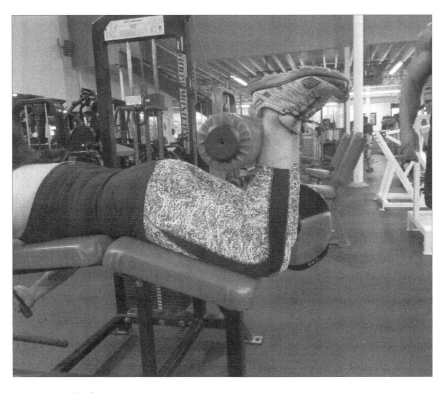

<u>Lying Leg Curl</u>

Curl up to the top, squeezing your hamstrings and buttocks, then lower your legs, stopping short of completely extending the knees.

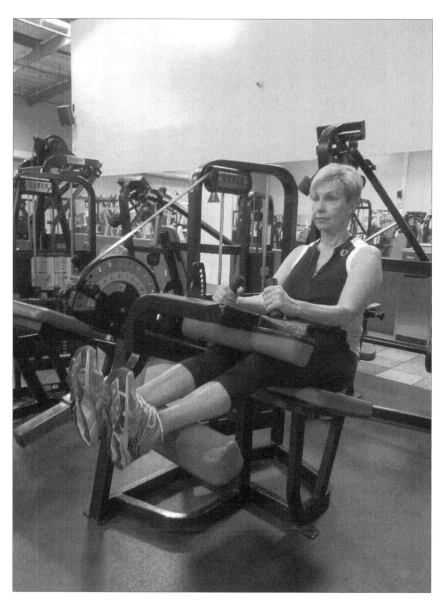

Seated Leg Curl

Have your back flat against the pad. Your knees are up against the bottom pad and your toes are pointed up and out.

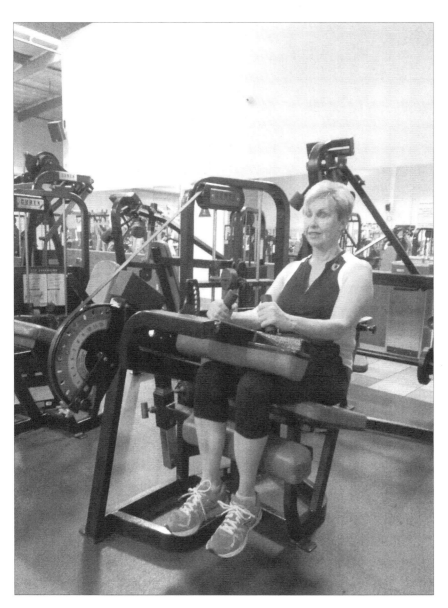

Seated Leg Curl

Pull down through your heels with your hamstrings, squeezing the hamstrings and glutes at the bottom. Return without letting the knees lock out.

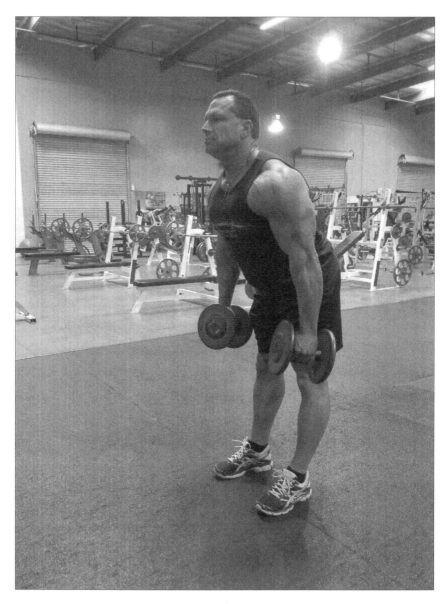

Stiff-Legged Dead Lifts

Your back is arched and hips out.

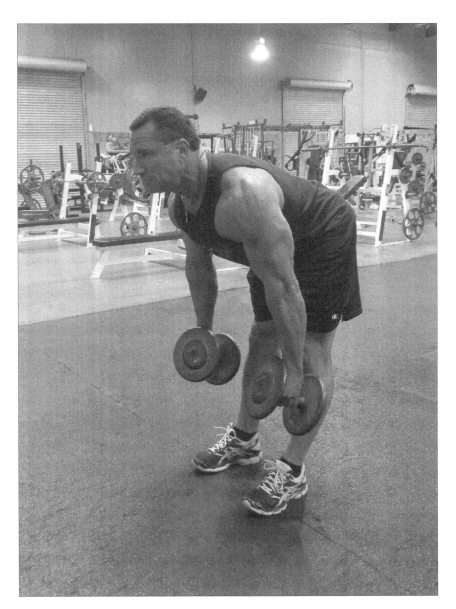

Stiff-Legged Dead Lifts

Keeping your back arched and shoulders back, bend over, pushing the hips out and letting the hamstrings take the weight down. Stretch as far as possible without losing the arch in your back. Then, using your hamstrings, pull your body up, stopping short of coming all the way up (this keeps the tension on the hamstrings).

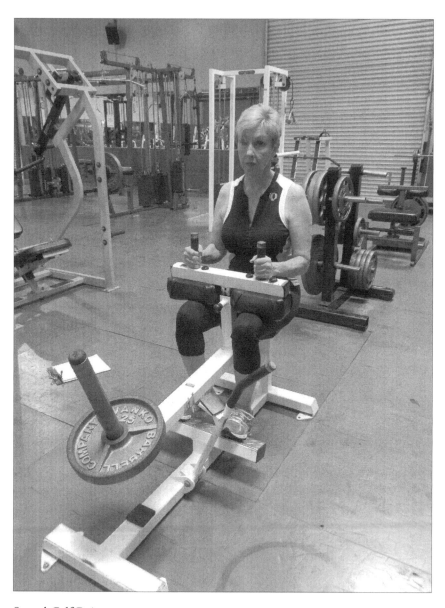

Seated Calf Raise

Have the pad above your knees and your toes slightly over the foot plate.

Seated Calf Raise

Push through the balls of your feet, going as high as possible. Then lower the feet and let the calves stretch at the bottom.

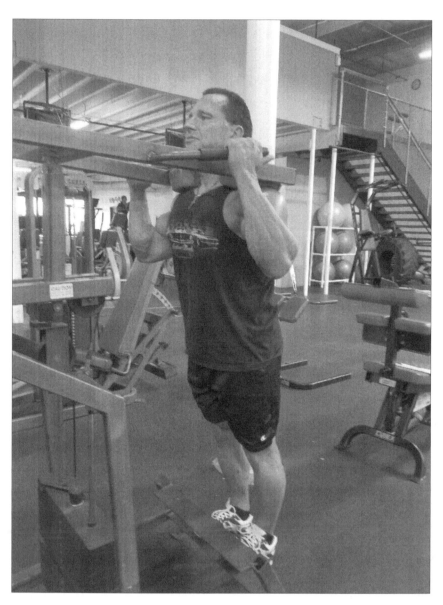

Standing Calf Raise

Keep your back and hips straight.

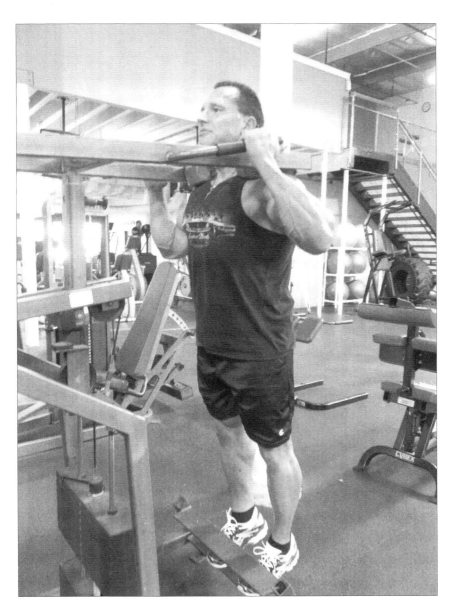

Standing Calf Raise

Push off the balls of your feet, coming up as high as you can, then lowering your feet, letting the calfs stretch at the bottom and then repeat.

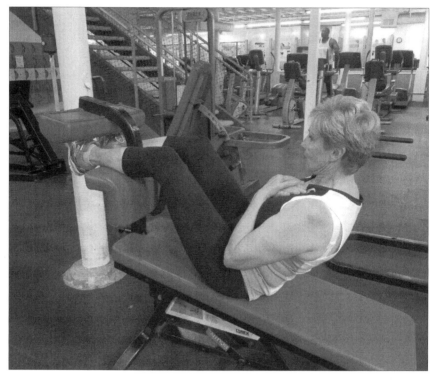

Ab Crunch

Start with your back curved and come up slowly, blowing your air out and squeezing your abs at the top.

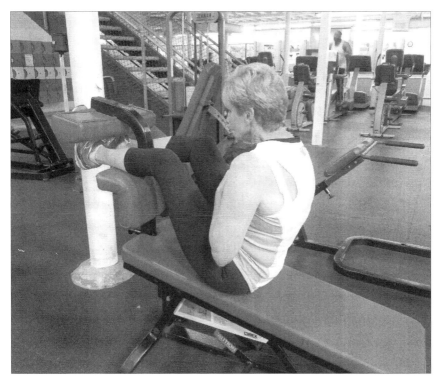

Ab Crunch

Return slowly, making sure to not go back too far or you'll feel the pressure increase on your back. This is a short, controlled movement.

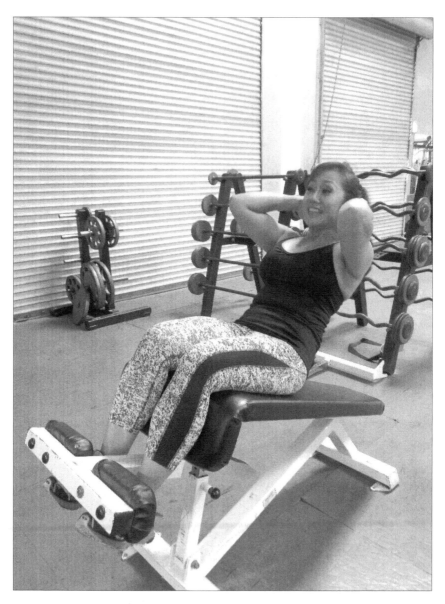

Ab Crunch Twist

This is the same as the regular crunch except you will twist at the top and squeeze the side of your abs.

*Never use your hand to pull yourself up.

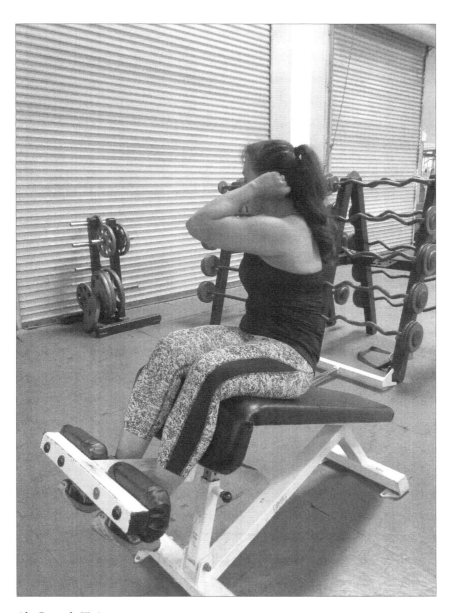

Ab Crunch Twist

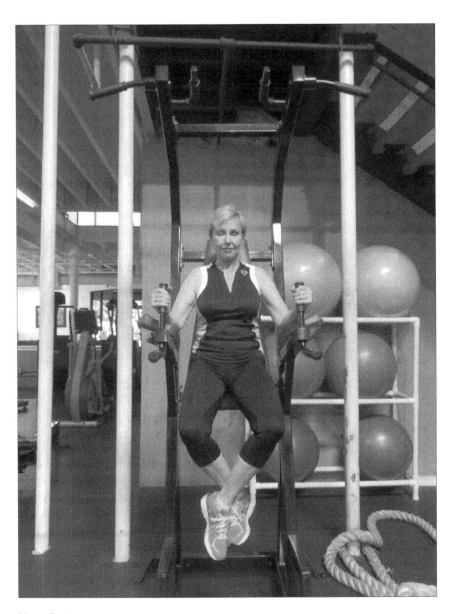

Knee Raises

With your back and elbows against the pad, cross your feet and pull your knees up as high as possible.

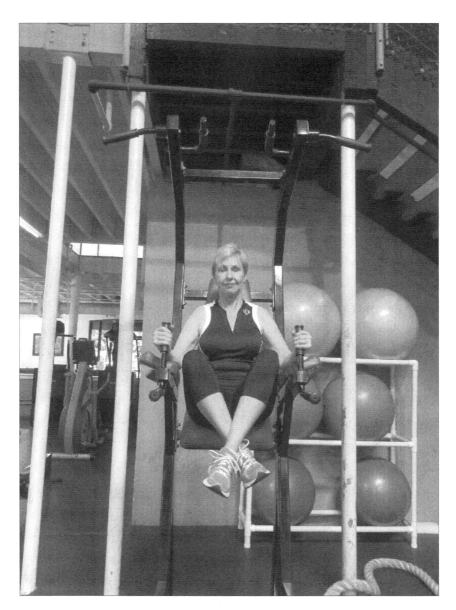

Knee Raises

At the top, blow out your air and squeeze your abs. Come down slowly and then go up again.

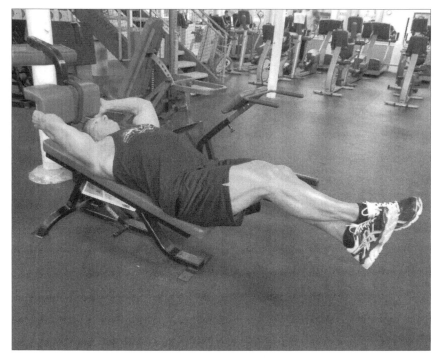

Leg Raises

These can be done on a flat bench or an angled bench.

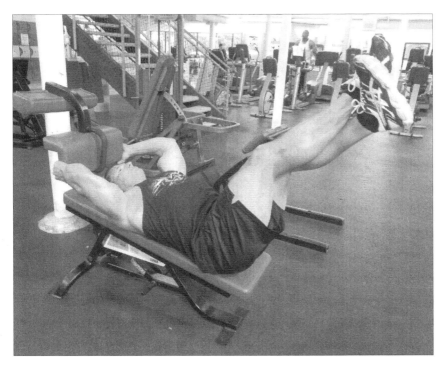

Leg Raises

While holding on to the bench, lift your legs up just over a 45-degree angle, pause and squeeze your abs. Then slowly lower your legs short of hitting 180 degrees (going lower adds pressure to your back).

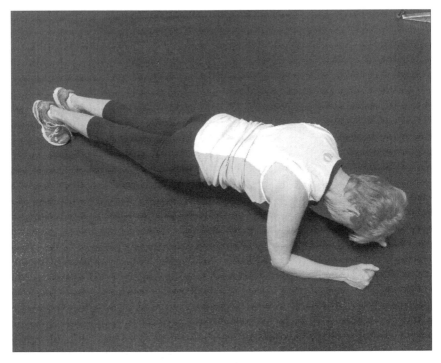

Plank

On your elbows and toes, with your arms at a 90-degree angle, your body is angled up but completely straight. While holding this position, squeeze your abs and glutes. Hold as long as you can and keep proper form.

Chapter 15

Cardio

Ve hear a lot of talk about all the different cardio exercises that exist. First, remember that any type of exercise that raises your heart rate over a period of time is a form of cardio. Going back to your weight training program, **once you have adapted your muscles and your mind to performing the exercises at a high level, every weight-training session will be a cardio session.**

"But what type of cardio is right for me?" is a question I get all the time. I have a simple, straightforward answer: "The one that you'll continue to do is the right one for you." Your body will adjust to cardio training faster than weight training. This means you will have to change or alter your cardio program more often. Now that I'm maintaining my body (not trying to get bigger, just staying fit), I use my strength training as a cardio session. I will keep my heart rate elevated throughout the entire workout.

In the beginning of your program, doing extra cardio will not only help your strength-training sessions and improve your fitness level, but will also help you lose body fat faster and reach your goals more quickly. Walking may be a great form of cardio for people in the beginning, but before long, you won't be able to get your heart rate high enough to get the optimal benefits. If you really enjoy walking, you'll have to look for steep hills or elevate the treadmill to increase your heart rate.

Start off easy with your cardio and gradually keep pushing yourself. There are different ways to increase your intensity. In the beginning, the easiest way is to increase your duration of time on cardio. The next option is to then increase your speed or resistance. For me, I like the elliptical machines. They allow me to get a high heart rate fairly easily without putting too much stress on my back, knees and feet. I usually have beginning clients start on a treadmill or bike to get used to doing cardio and then increase their intensity or move them to the elliptical.

If this is new to you, I recommend starting with 10-15 minutes the first week or two. Then start increasing the time and the intensity. If your goal is to drop a lot of body fat, you will want to work up to 45 minutes of cardio. Once you can do 45 minutes of cardio, you don't need to go any longer. Rather, work on increasing your intensity. If you're just looking to get in shape, I'd keep the time between 20-30 minutes. This will help you from getting burned out on cardio or dreading long cardio sessions.

There are two games I play to help me pass the time while doing cardio. First, every two minutes, I'll go up 1-2 levels until I'm struggling, and then I'll go down one level every two minutes and repeat. This increases the intensity and seems to help the time go by a little faster. The second is a more advanced type of cardio. I'll go "all out" for two minutes, then I'll go easy for about 60-90 seconds, and then repeat that again for six rounds. As your cardio improves, you can increase your speed or resistance during your high-intensity rounds. There are many variations you can do to mix it up. Find what you like and keep pushing it.

The next question is what to do first: cardio or weights? I could argue both sides of this, but the bottom line is picking the order that's best for you. It's getting them both done that counts. For me, I like strength training first and cardio second. It takes more mental focus for my strength training, whereas with cardio, I can hit "autopilot" and push through it. Some people prefer to do cardio first to help them warm up and get them ready to do their strength training. Give both a try and see what order you prefer—or mix them up, too.

If you're training 2-3 days per week, you have another option. You could do cardio on your off days or on your training days. Again, pick what's going to fit your lifestyle the best. I prefer to do my cardio with my training so I can spend more time with my family and have days I don't have to go to the gym.

I enjoy riding my bike outside. It's a good change of pace and something different. I'm not a racing or distance cyclist, so I'm not going to reach the same heart rate levels I would if I were in the gym. I love hiking and biking, but those are activities I use to supplement my cardio, not replace it.

Chapter 16

An Overview of Nutrition

Nutrition is a topic on which everyone has an opinion, and an area in which everyone is trying to cut corners to get faster and easier results. The truth is, nutrition isn't that complicated, but it is very much misunderstood. Again, with good reason because large companies want you to buy their quick-fix, easy-results types of products or sell you meals and shakes that, once you stop consuming, if you did drop any body fat, it will generally come right back. I tell my clients that nutrition is like simple math: 1+1+1=3.

▸ The first "1" is **the right type of food.**
▸ The second "1" is **adding the right amount of food to your diet.**
▸ The third "1" is **eating at the right times.**

They add up to "3," which is dropping body fat, adding lean muscle and feeling better than ever!

We all want a quick fix, but one doesn't exist. It took time to put on the body fat; it will take some time to take it off. The key is to take it off the right way and keep it off forever! When you try to change this simple formula, you may lose weight in the beginning, but you're setting yourself up for failure in the end. That's why so many people struggle with fluctuating weight. Don't be frustrated with your past attempts. Follow my simple plan and you'll drop body fat a little more slowly than with an extreme fad diet, but you'll continue to drop it while reshaping your body to look and feel better than ever. Plus, since it's not a program, but rather, a change in your lifestyle, you'll not only keep off the fat you lost, but you'll also continue to keep improving as you go—even after you've hit your goals.

Looking back over the last seven decades, **what group has been the most successful in dropping body fat and improving lean muscle mass? Bodybuilders!** What's their secret? **They don't try to cut any corners.** They train hard, do their cardio exercise, eat properly and adjust their food to increase fat loss. No magic or gimmicks, just simple addition and consistency.

When I was competing, I would have to go to an extreme to get my body fat down to around 4 percent. The good news is there's no reason for anyone who's not competing to do that. **You can reach your goals the same way we do, but you won't have to go through the extreme parts of the program.** You have to trust me on this: Once you're on the program for a while, it actually gets easier and easier to follow it and improve. The beginning is always the most difficult. You just need to stay focused and committed to your program in the beginning and you'll get there.

Let's start with the first rule about nutrition and fat loss that I go over with my clients. Just like the marathon example, we tend to go from eating poorly to starting on a strict diet in one step and then wonder why it's so difficult and we fail. Of course, you just tried to run 26 miles on your first day! **You didn't put on the body fat in one week; it's not going to come off in one week.**

Another mistake is trying to cut meals or cut calories too quickly. Ideally, you want to eat a complete meal every 3-4 hours. If you're only eating two meals a day right now, your metabolism is going to be slow and you probably won't lose any body fat. **When your body is deprived of food, it will want to hold onto the stored fat instead of burning it for fuel.** Your body doesn't know when you're going to eat again, so it wants to hold onto the fat. If this is you, then you'll want to add in one meal while making all of your meals smaller. Don't go from two meals a day to six, as it's too drastic of a change. We want your body to adjust to your program.

We also tend to eat way too much at every meal. **If you control your portion sizes, you will feel better, burn more fat, and your body will run more efficiently.** Six meals a day may seem like a lot, but again, start slowly. Add in one meal at a time and slowly work your way up to 5-6 meals per day. You will turn your body into a fat-burning machine. It's normal to think, "I'm eating three times per day and not losing weight, and you want me to add 2-3 more meals? I'll gain even more!" That's not true if you do it right. For example, when I would start getting ready for a show, I would be eating three times per day.

As I got closer to my competition, I would adjust my protein/carb/fat ratios, which would slightly lower my overall caloric intake. Then I would actually increase my meals to seven times per day. As I made my adjustments, I'd go up to eight, then nine meals per day. Granted, my training intensity was very high, and the food I was eating was very restrictive, but I ate nine times per day and dropped body fat faster than ever. I was rarely hungry because, by the time I was, it was time to eat again. I am not saying I didn't have any craving to eat something off my diet, but I was full after every meal. There is no reason to go to this extreme, however, and I don't recommend it. You will adjust to eating 5-6 meals per day and you should feel full and have plenty of energy.

Now, for me to maintain where I'm at, I eat 5-7 meals a day. The variance comes from my day and the size of my meals. You should notice that as you add meals, you should be hungry at every meal time because your body is running more efficiently and is looking for the energy to keep it running smoothly.

I have many clients who, in the beginning, didn't eat breakfast. They'd say they're not hungry when they get up. I convince them to just **eat something with a little protein every morning for two weeks**. Every time, by the end of the two weeks, they are amazed that every morning they wake up hungry. Again, it's because your body is functioning better and burning more fat.

Snacking

We don't realize how many extra empty calories we consume by snacking. This will be hard at first, but you will get used to it. **You don't snack! Period!** If you feel you have to snack, you need to check two things. First, did you eat enough at your last meal, or is it time for you to eat again? Most snack food will completely sabotage your program. Your meals are designed to keep you full longer and your blood-sugar levels stable. This will help you burn more body fat for energy while making your body healthier. Keeping stable blood-sugar levels not only helps you drop body fat and increase lean muscle, it's the best way to prevent type 2 diabetes.

There are a few exceptions to snacking, which I call "mini meals."

What's a mini meal? A mini meal is a small, healthy meal that would be one of your daily meals. These are quick, easy things to eat to keep your metabolism going and your blood-sugar levels stable. This is a meal that's eaten at one point during the day—you don't continue to keep eating and prolonging the snack. It's a quick meal and you're done. Since it's usually a lower-calorie meal, designed to hold you over until the next meal, you can eat again in about two hours rather than in 3-4 hours. These mini meals help keep you from cheating and/or from going too long between meals. If you go too long between meals, you will become overly hungry and want to not only eat bad food, but more of it.

Your main goal of eating this way is to create an easily sustainable lifestyle change that you can live with forever. Again, the first few weeks will be the hardest, but after that, your body and mind will adjust to your new program. It will get easier and easier the longer you go. Eventually, you'll reach a point where you won't even feel like you're on an eating plan—it will just be natural because that's what your body wants. When you do eat something bad, you're likely to feel somewhat sick because your body isn't used to eating those things anymore.

I ask all my new clients to completely give up fast food for one month. I tell them that after that one month, they can go and get whatever and as much as they want (I always hear about how much they miss it and I encourage them). It's just one month, and then they can have all they want. When their month is up, I hear about how they can't wait to go eat their favorite fast food—that they can already taste it. Over 90 percent of the time when they get their old, favorite food, it tastes terrible to them and they end up throwing it away. They're amazed they actually miss their healthy food, and shocked at how bad their old, favorite foods tasted. Many even feel sick after they have finished their old, fast-food meal. Your tastes and preferences will change for the better—it just takes time and consistency.

One of the favorite diet questions I get—and I get it all the time—is about specific vegetables. People tell me they're on a new eating program and they're not eating any peas, carrots or corn in order to lose body fat. Sorry if I laugh a little, but I then ask them, "Have you ever heard of anyone, I mean anyone, complain that they've gained too much body fat because they can't stop eating peas, carrots or corn?" They think for a second and laugh with me when they realize how crazy that is. Okay, those foods do contain more sugar than other fibrous green vegetables, but in 25 years, I've never met anyone who had this as their main problem. It's the dessert, snacks and junk we eat every day without even thinking about it. Plus, when you're eating your peas, carrots and corn, you should be having them with a good, low-fat protein that will slow down how fast that little bit of sugar gets into your bloodstream.

Don't over-think it, but at the same time, think everything though. I had a client tell me that she had gone to dinner and was so proud of herself for not eating her baked potato in order to help keep her carbs down. She then went on to tell me how the chocolate cake was to die for. Really? **Eat the potato and don't eat the cake!**

It's popular now to cut carbs out of your eating program for fast weight loss. Although that will help you lose weight, know that in the first two weeks, half of the weight you will lose is water weight. Cutting out carbs will work, but it simply isn't a sustainable plan. When I was at the toughest part of my pre-contest diet, I'd cut out all carbs except vegetables for only three days, then I'd have a high-carb day. This would do a few things: It would replace the stored carbs in the muscle that I had depleted, and it would help keep my metabolism running faster. Also, it would give me back some sanity and make me feel as if I had gotten a short break from my diet. Doing this also helped me get through the tough days, knowing I had another carb day coming soon. Remember, that was for an extreme phase of my program. You want to have a program that not only gives you great results, but also allows you to live a happy lifestyle that's not about food all the time.

Another mistake I see people make is skipping a meal if they have eaten or are going to eat an unhealthy one. Doing these things will set yourself up for failure, as you'll become overly hungry and repeat the same cycle. If you eat an unhealthy meal, don't get down on yourself. Just get back to the plan, and in 3-4 hours, have your next healthy meal. Even if you're not hungry, eat it anyway and get back on track.

From my personal experience, if you're craving something unhealthy, "tough it out" or have a mini meal. **If you're craving something very particular and that craving persists, go ahead and have it and then get right back on track.** I've found that, too many times in the beginning, if I had a very specific craving, I'd do everything to try to avoid it and then end up eating it anyway. So you're better off just eating it and then getting right back to your plan. If this is happening often, then you need to look at your program. You're probably not getting something right and need to make an adjustment.

Alcohol is another big problem some people have. I would say give it up until you reach your goals, but that isn't going to work for some people. If you're not going to give it up, let's make a few smart choices. Try to cut back the times and the amount you drink. Also, if you're going to drink, make sure you're not adding any extra calories to your drink. Many drinks are full of sugar along with the alcohol, and that will stop your program flat. I had one client who drank four margaritas a day. I had her cut back to 2-3 drinks only on 2-3 days per week and to have the tequila with soda water or on the rocks to cut out the extra sugar. She did that and dropped 20 pounds of fat over three months.

Also, if you're drinking alcohol, don't snack. Have your meal before and know in advance your meal for after. You have to be conscious of this. It's all too easy after a few drinks to end up eating poorly. If you plan it out, you will be able to stay on track with your program. Another good idea is to drink extra water while you're drinking alcohol. This will help you from becoming dehydrated and can slow down how much you drink.

Another pitfall is going out to eat. If possible, tell the waiter not to bring bread to the table. It's too easy to fill up on bread and add extra calories to your day. I always like to have a glass of water before a meal. This helps me fill up faster so I don't overeat, and it's extremely important to stay hydrated for losing body fat. If you have a salad, ask for a low-calorie dressing on the side. This way, you can control how much you use on your salad. If you like to get appetizers, go for some grilled or fresh vegetables or a lean, non-fried protein. If the dinner comes with sides, I normally ask for extra vegetables instead or one starchy carb, of which I'll only eat half. Sometimes I'll get extra protein. You want to eat healthy and avoid getting dessert. It might be tough at first to pass on the desserts, but you'll be happier walking out of dinner when you do. Following these tips will help you stay on track with your program and continue to move forward.

As a general rule, don't drink your calories! This means no sugary drinks, such as sodas and juices, and watch what you're putting in your coffee. Don't add these extra calories; they'll completely stop your body from burning fat. Healthy juices are very popular now. Be careful to get ones that consist mostly of vegetables and have one or two fresh fruits—not fruit juice. Also, protein shakes are a good, quick way to get in a meal, but again, be careful of what goes into them.

What about fruit? Yes, fruit contains sugar, but one piece of fruit or a cup of berries is good for you; and remember, you're eating it *with* a meal, not as a snack. When you're eating fruit with a good, lean protein and a little bit of fat, it will slow down how fast the sugar is released into your bloodstream, helping you keep your blood-sugar levels stabilized. This will help lead you to prolonged, stable energy while increasing your fat-burning potential.

Sugar

Without getting too technical, I believe it's important to understand how and what sugar does to your body. And, hey, **it's usually the main reason we gain weight or are unable to lose weight.** When we eat any type of carb, our bodies break it down into glucose that then goes into your bloodstream. Simple sugars and/or processed carbs significantly and quickly increase your blood-sugar levels. This tells the pancreas to release insulin, which does two things: It tells the body to stop using fat for energy and to put the sugar somewhere. When your blood-sugar levels are too high, you will release more insulin than your body needs and it will pull too much glucose out of your blood, causing your blood-sugar levels to drop below normal. This will make your body crave more sugar to get its levels back up to normal. It's a vicious cycle. **If your muscle and liver glycogen levels are full, your body will simply take the extra glucose out of your blood and convert it to fat.** This is why it is so important to maintain steady blood-sugar levels. This is also why you don't want to snack between meals. Your body is running off of stored fat. When you snack, you shut down the fat-burning process and raise your blood-sugar levels.

One More Tip: Water

You need to make sure you're drinking enough water. Water will help you avoid dehydration, which slows down your body's fat-burning potential. Water also helps to remove toxins from your body. If you're not getting enough water, you may feel tired. This is from a reduction of oxygen to your muscles. It can also affect your joints. Personally, if I forget to drink enough water, I get a headache, but after 15 minutes of getting in my water, the headache is gone. **Drinking water before and after you eat can help you feel fuller and eat less.** It is commonly recommended that you drink eight, 8-oz. glasses of water per day. If you're training hard and/or it's hot, you're going to have to increase the amount you drink. **Drinking more water will not make you hold water—it will actually help you flush out your body, making you look and feel better.**

Chapter 17

How to Put Your Meals Together

L et's start with the basics. The food you eat is broken down into three categories:

1. **Proteins**
2. **Carbs**
3. **Fats**

I'll give you a simple list of these foods to pick from to complete your food program. Even though foods are listed under certain categories, they will still have some amounts of the other nutrients in them. For example, red meat is a protein, but will also have some fat in it. Peanut butter is a fat, but it also contains both proteins and carbs.

If you're just embarking upon a healthy eating program, start at the beginning. No need to jump ahead or try anything crazy. If you can eat healthy, balanced meals and avoid junk food, you're well on your way. Once your body has adjusted to your new eating program, you can make some changes as you go. The advantage to this is that it will be both mentally and physically easier on you to adjust to your new program. Also, when you start making these changes, your body will adapt to them better and you'll continue to get results. Another advantage to making small adjustments to your plan is, if you feel off or it's not working, you can look at what your last adjustment was and fix it by changing your food ratios, whereas, if you had made multiple changes all at once, you wouldn't be sure which one of the changes was causing the problem.

One personal example was when I was preparing for my first show. My diet got to a point where my carbs were very low. I noticed my energy was dropping way too fast. When I went back and looked at my food intake, I realized I wasn't consuming enough fat for my energy to make up for the cut in carbs. Once I increased my fat intake just enough, I felt better right away.

Step No. 1

For each meal, you want to pick a "good" carb and a lean protein. To start, I'd pick an equal amount of carbs and protein, so **50 percent of your calories are from carbs and 50 percent are from protein.** It's always a great idea to add in some vegetables and/or a salad with your meal. These will help you feel and stay full. Make sure to not add too many extra calories to your salad.

Your goal is to eat 5-6 small meals. If you're not there now, that's okay; make your meals smaller and add an extra one in until you get there. This is an example of a meal plan I'd start a client on:

For a Woman:
▸ 20-30 grams of protein per meal
▸ 20-30 grams of carbs per meal
▸ 5 grams of fat per meal

This is *not* counting grams of food from vegetables and salad.

This would be repeated 4-5 times per day and would be between 820-1,425 calories for the 4-5 meals, depending on the size and number of meals. I usually go by the grams of protein, carbs and fat, not including the calories from vegetables. This makes it easier to follow and to know your ratios. This is a 50/50 protein-to-carb ratio. In this phase, we try to keep the fat to a minimum.

For a Man:
▸ 40-50 grams of protein per meal
▸ 40-50 grams of carbs per meal
▸ 10 grams of fat per meal

You'll see these are the same ratios as the woman's, but larger numbers. The overall calorie count could be between 2,050-2,762, again, depending on the number and size of the meals.

Depending on body size and activity level, the grams will be adjusted for both women and men.

This isn't everyone's starting point, but it's a good place to start if you're not sure. You will have to gauge your weight and activity level and adjust your ratios from there. If I had a female client who wanted to lose body fat and tone up, this is one example of the plan I would put together—keeping in mind that everyone is different and we make adjustments to those differences as we go.

Each phase would last 10-20 days depending on body-fat loss and how the individual was feeling and performing on the program.

The first number is always protein, second is carbs and third is fat.

Phase 1:
30/30/5: 4 meals per day, adjustment to eating 4 times per day

Phase 2:
25/25/5: 5 meals per day, increasing training and meal frequency

Phase 3:
30/20/5: 5-6 meals per day, increasing intensity and protein intake and slightly dropping carb intake

Phase 4:
35/15/5-8: 5-6 times per day

Phase 5:
35/15/5-10: first 3 meals
35/0/5-10: last 2-3 meals; major cutting phase

This will usually get my clients to their main goal. With each phase, we increase the intensity of our training and cardio. If you want to continue to a more extreme phase, you can, although it is not usually needed (some clients like to test and push themselves to see what they can achieve).

Then we have Phase 6.

Phase 6:
35-40/0/5-10: all meals for two days (again, still eating a lot of green veggies)

On the third day, you would have a carb day and it would consist of the following:

30/30-40/5: *all meals except the last meal,* which would go back to **35-40/0/5-10.**

Then repeat the same cycle: two days no carbs and then one carb day.

Phase 7 is the same as Phase 6:

35-40/0/5-10: but you're going three days with only veggies, then having the same carb day on the fourth day, then repeating.

This is a difficult eating program, but one that gets amazing results. After finishing a Phase 6 and/or 7, you need to be careful not to over-eat. You've gone extreme; have your plan ready for when you're done. I usually have clients going back to Phase 3 or 4, or a combination of both. There are many variations of what you can do. This is to give you one idea. See what works best for you.

The following are simple lists of proteins, carbs and fats:

PROTEINS			
Ahi	Monk Fish	Filet Mignon	Deli Chicken
Bass	Oysters	Flank Steak	Deli Turkey
Catfish	Perch	London Broil	Egg White only
Clams	Salmon	Round Steak	Egg Whole
Cod	Scallops	Top Sirloin	Lean Lamb
Crab	Shark	Egg Beaters	Low-Fat Cottage Cheese
Flounder	Snapper	Protein Shake	Low-Fat Milk
Haddock	Swordfish	Protein Powder	Non-Fat Milk
Halibut	Tuna in Water	93% Ground Turkey	Pork Tenderloin
Lobster	Yellow Tail	98% Free Deli Ham	Turkey Breast
Mahi Mahi	93% Lean Hamburger	Chicken Breast	

COMPLEX CARBS		
7-Grain Bread	Multi-Grain Bread	Squash
Beans: Black, Pinto, Kidney	Oatmeal	Sweet Potato
Corn Tortillas	Potato	Whole Wheat Bread
Couscous	Quinoa	Yam
Cream of Rice	Low-Fat Refried Beans	Low-Sugar Cereal
Cream of Wheat	Rice	Pasta

FRUITS (Simple Carbs)	
Apple	Nectarine
Apricot	Orange
Blackberries	Peach
Blueberries	Pear
Cherries	Raspberries
Grapefruit	Strawberries
Grapes	Watermelon

VEGETABLES				
Alfalfa Sprouts	Cabbage	Cucumber	Mushrooms	Radish
Artichoke	Carrots	Eggplant	Okra	Snow Peas
Asparagus	Cauliflower	Green Beans	Onion	Spinach
Broccoli	Celery	Leeks	Peas	Tomato
Brussels Sprouts	Corn	Lettuce	Peppers	Zucchini

FATS		
Peanut butter	Butter	Extra Virgin Olive Oil
Almond Butter	Flaxseed Oil	Peanuts
Avocado	Odu's Oil	Almonds

Chapter 18

How to Stick to Your Nutritional Program

Τhis definitely is the area in which most of us struggle. How do you stay on your eating program? The two keys are **preparation** and **planning**! Starting with preparation: The easiest mistake to make is not having any food ready to eat when you get hungry. This is when we make simple and quick choices of what to eat, and it's usually the wrong type of food. The best way to avoid this is by **always having at home all the food you need—including backup food—for all your meals.** I pre-cook my chicken for the week and cut up a variety of different veggies and have them mixed in a bowl, ready to go. Also, I pre-cook rice and/or potatoes so they're ready at a moment's notice. This way, if you don't have time to cook a full meal, you can quickly mix the protein, carbs and veggies together in just a few minutes and you have your healthy meal. Another prep I do for my meals is to pre-portion them and have them made up so all I have to do is heat them up. This is great for taking food to work or being on-the-go. Since I'm on the road most of the day, I always have a few pre-made protein shakes and some almonds with me. If I run out of food or forget a meal, that's what I'll have instead. Not only will it hold me over until my next meal, it's quick and easy and it will keep me from stopping and getting food I shouldn't have.

For my planning, I think of how many meals I will need for the next workday. I'll put them together in the evening and have them ready to go when I wake up in the morning. Another advantage to this is your portions are already divided up and you won't overeat.

As I previously mentioned, one area in which I see many people struggle is going out to eat. You can and should go out to eat, but again, plan ahead for not only where you are going, but what you are going to eat. I had a client who, for his business, had to go out for lunch or dinner almost every day. To help him continue to drop body fat, we would find out ahead of time where he'd be dining. If we could control the place where they went to eat, it was even better. I'd get copies of the menus from every restaurant he would generally go to, and we'd review the menu the day before. I'd show him the best entrées to get and what to definitely stay away from. Since he knew ahead of time what he would be ordering, he would order without even looking at the menu. This helped him to stay on track and not make poor decisions. These things aren't hard to do, but they won't just happen by themselves. You need to work on this and perfect it for yourself. You can do it—it just takes a little extra time and planning on your part. The results will be well worth the time invested.

Chapter 19

Preparation for the Gym

This is a must for anyone beginning a strength-training program. Before you go to the gym, you need to start preparing for your workout. If possible, **try to have a meal approximately 90 minutes before you train.** This will give you energy to train and your stomach time to empty so the blood can be used for the muscles—not for digestion.

Everyone is different. Some people might feel nauseous if they have anything before training, so their meal may have to be smaller and eaten two hours before training. You'll have to try some different options and see what makes your body feel the best. Personally, I can't go to the gym if I'm really hungry, so I'll make a small, light protein drink to help me get through it.

Now that your body is fueled up, you need to go over your training routine for the day. Know what muscles you are going to train and what exercises you're going to perform. Know what order you're going to do them in and also what style and techniques you're going to use. Is it going to be a heavy day, a higher-rep day, supersets, drop sets, slow rep day and/or a combination of multiple styles? I always have a game plan in place before I get to the gym. This helps you from becoming lax and doing the same workout the same way and hitting plateaus. Plus, it will keep the workouts exciting and fun. I also plan for some flexibility in my workout. For example, if it's busy and the exercise you're going to do next is taken, have a backup exercise in mind. You don't want to waste time and diminish your workout by waiting around. Stay focused and on your mission!

In the beginning, when you get home, write down some notes on the exercises, styles and rep ranges you performed. You can look back at your workouts, which will help you better plan your future.

Another part of planning your workouts is to write down the days and times you will be training and try your best to stick to what you write down. This will help you from skipping days or putting your training off until "later," when it generally won't happen.

After your training, you want to consume a high-protein, moderate-carb meal to help your muscles recover. I struggle to get in a solid meal after I train, so I will usually make a protein shake with greens and berries for my post-training meal. Have some backup meals ready and see what your body feels like eating. **Just get that meal in within an hour of training.**

Chapter 20

Conclusion

Now you have the knowledge of how to do and set up everything in your program to reach all your goals.

- Write down all your goals.
- You will be successful!
- Get mentally prepared for your program from every aspect.
- Write out everything from training days, times, styles and techniques, exercises, cardio and meals.

Simply follow the 4 Rules of Training:

- No. 1: Consistency
- No. 2: Mentally focus on the muscle, not on the weight
- No. 3: Proper form
- No. 4: Perform each set until full muscle fatigue

You will enjoy watching your body change and become leaner and stronger than ever before.

Good luck! Stay committed and reach new levels of fitness!

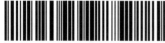

Made in the USA
San Bernardino, CA
15 April 2015